YOUR FEET

Questions
you
have
...Answers
you
need

Other Books in This Series
From the People's Medical Society

YOUR FEET

Questions you have ...Answers you need

By Sandra Salmans

≡People's Medical Society®

Allentown, Pennsylvania

The People's Medical Society is a nonprofit consumer health organization dedicated to the principles of better, more responsive and less expensive medical care. Organized in 1983, the People's Medical Society puts previously unavailable medical information into the hands of consumers so that they can make informed decisions about their own health care.

Membership in the People's Medical Society is $20 a year and includes a subscription to the *People's Medical Society Newsletter.* For information, write to the People's Medical Society, 462 Walnut Street, Allentown, PA 18102, or call 610-770-1670.

This and other People's Medical Society publications are available for quantity purchase at discount. Contact the People's Medical Society for details.

© 1998 by the People's Medical Society
Printed in the United States of America

Library of Congress Cataloging-in-Publication Data
Salmans, Sandra.
 Your feet : questions you have, answers you need /
by Sandra Salmans.
   p. cm.
 Includes bibliographical references and index.
 ISBN 1-882606-40-X
 1. Foot—Care and hygiene—Miscellanea. 2. Foot—Wounds and injuries—Miscellanea. 3. Foot—Diseases—Miscellanea.
4. Foot—Diseases—Popular works. 5. Self-care, Health. I. Title.
RD563.S23 1998
617.5'85—dc21   98-3354
                   CIP

1 2 3 4 5 6 7 8 9 0
First printing, July 1998

CONTENTS

INTRODUCTION

Probably no part of our bodies takes more abuse than
our feet. From childhood to old age, our feet are our
primary mode of transportation, carrying our bodies from
here to there, in rain and snow, up and down stairs, with
no shoes or tight shoes, with nary a rest. No wonder
most people suffer some type of foot problem. Whether
blisters or corns, bunions or hammertoes, the maladies
of our feet are large in number. And many of them can
be debilitating.

Feet have also become an industry. Whole sections
of drugstores are devoted to our feet. Shelves are loaded
with ointments, inserts, clippers and braces. A bevy of
health care practitioners concentrates on our feet. And
every major shoe manufacturer tells us that it's developed
the perfect vehicle for our feet.

Yet, as big a problem as feet can be, most of us know
very little about them. From their complex structure to
the strategies for keeping them in shape, we're basically
podiatrically ignorant! And that is precisely why we
developed this book.

Your Feet: Questions You Have ... Answers You Need
is the one-stop guide to your feet. From what can go
wrong to how to prevent a problem, this book answers
all your questions. In fact, we've written the book in our
popular question-and-answer format to make everything
you need to know easy to find and understand.

Like all People's Medical Society books, *Your Feet:
Questions You Have ... Answers You Need* is meant to
empower. The more you know about your health and
medical treatments, the better your chances of having
fewer problems. And knowing what can go wrong with
your feet and what can be done about it is essential.

And you should know something else about this book.
What you're about to read is information that comes
directly from the medical literature. It is not opinion or
just one practitioner's approach to a problem. Author
Sandra Salmans has scoured the studies, interviewed the
leading experts and translated the medical gobbledygook
to ensure that what you find in these pages is the most
accurate and up-to-date information available. We're con-
fident that what you need to know about foot problems
will be found between these covers.

As the nation's largest nonprofit consumer health
advocacy organization, our only goal is to help you be a
more informed and better health care consumer. I'm con-
fident that this book will go a long way in accomplishing
that goal.

CHARLES B. INLANDER
President
People's Medical Society

YOUR FEET

**Questions
you
have
...Answers
you
need**

Terms printed in boldface can be found in the glossary, beginning on page 165. Only the first mention of the word in the text will be boldfaced.

We have tried to use male and female pronouns in an egalitarian manner throughout the book. Any imbalance in usage has been in the interest of readability.

1 FEET FIRST

Q: Let's get to the bottom of it: What is the basic structure of the foot?

A: The foot is a complicated and masterful piece of bioengineering. The American Podiatric Medical Association (APMA), which tends to wax lyrical on the subject, compares it with a finely tuned race car or a space shuttle—a vehicle whose function dictates its design and structure. More prosaically, we'd say that the foot is an extraordinarily flexible structure that, for its size, has an amazing ability to withstand crushing impact and provide powerful propulsion.

For a start, each foot contains at least 26 bones. Some experts count the bones differently and come up with 28. And children's feet appear to contain even more bones, because the bones don't completely fuse before the age of 20 years or so. In any event, the bones in your two feet together make up about one-quarter of all the bones in your entire body. Each foot also contains 33 joints; a network of more than 100 **tendons** (fibrous cords of tissue that connect muscle to bone), muscles and **ligaments** (tough, fibrous tissues that connect bones to each other); and innumerable blood vessels and nerves.

Q: What are the important bones in the foot?

A: For anatomical purposes, the foot can be sub-divided into three sections: the rearfoot, the midfoot and the forefoot. The rearfoot consists of just the

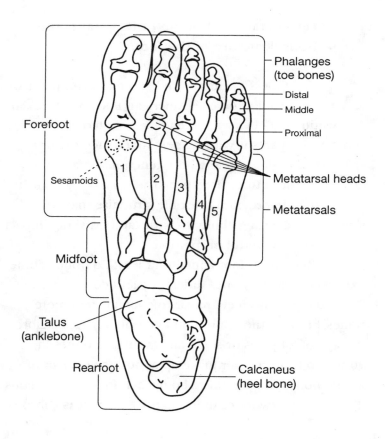

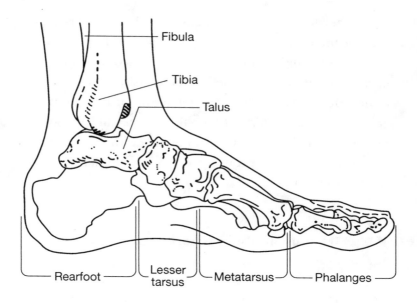

 anklebone, or **talus**, and the heel bone, or **calcaneus**—
the largest bone in your foot. These two bones connect
to form the **subtalar joint**, which allows you to rotate
your foot at the ankle. The talus also connects with the
tibia—the inner and larger bone of the two bones of the
leg below the knee—and the **fibula**—the outer and
smaller of the two bones.

In the midfoot, there are five irregular bones called the
tarsals, or, collectively, the lesser tarsus. Together these
form the arch that gives your foot its spring (and often
contributes to foot problems).

Finally, there's the forefoot. Connected to the tarsals
are the five long **metatarsal** bones that bear more than
half your weight as you walk and put pressure on the
balls of your feet. At the other end, each metatarsal connects to a **phalanx** (pl., phalanges), or toe bone. Foot

care specialists refer to the metatarsals by number—
one for the bone connecting to the big toe, five for the
bone connecting to the small toe. Toes two through five
each have three bones. The big toe consists of only two
bones. However, beneath the metatarsal for the big toe
are the two **sesamoids**, the smallest bones in the foot.
Despite their size, they serve a key function, enabling
muscles to move your foot up and down and letting
the big toe move.

Q: **What do all those tendons, muscles and ligaments do?**

A: They hold the foot together and provide the
extraordinary flexibility that allows ballet dancers
to stand *en pointe* and you to walk and run. The tendons
attach the muscle to the bone and transmit the force that
the muscles exert. The 20 or so different muscles help
the foot keep its shape, holding the bones in position and
tugging on the tendons, allowing the foot to move. The
ligaments hold the tendons in place.

The largest and strongest tendon in your foot is the
famous **Achilles tendon**, which runs from the middle
of the back of the leg to the heel bone. It's named after
the Greek hero whose mother, myth has it, tried to make
him immortal by dipping him into the river Styx. But
because she held on to his ankle, he remained vulnerable
in that one spot and was wounded fatally there during
the Trojan War. Your Achilles tendon won't kill you, but
it can cause you problems, as discussed in chapter 2.

Q: Are there any ligaments that are equally important?

A: In this book, you'll be reading a lot about what is the longest ligament in the foot, and possibly the strongest ligament in the entire body—the **plantar fascia**. It runs along the sole, from the heel to the ball of the foot, and supports the arch. When you stand, the plantar fascia stretches like a rubber band from your heel to your big toe, absorbing most of the downward pressure; when you raise your foot, the ligament loosens and curves upward into your arch.

In addition to the plantar fascia, there are two important groups of ligaments that hold your foot stable and allow it to move up and down (and, like the plantar fascia, are particularly susceptible to injury, as discussed in chapter 2). These are the **medial** ligaments, on the inside of the foot, and the **lateral** ligaments, on the outside of the foot.

Q: Is there anything else I should know about the structure of the foot?

A: The bare-bones anatomy doesn't begin to describe the enormous variation in feet—in width, height of arches, and shape of toes and other areas, all of which can contribute to foot problems. Arches, for example, differ in their **pronation**, or how they flatten when you step down. Normally, your foot strikes the ground with the back of the heel first and then rolls toward the ball or the metatarsal area. As it does, your entire heel comes to rest on the ground, and your arch lowers a little. If your arch pronates too much or too little, you can have problems, as discussed in chapter 2.

Q: **Earlier you mentioned the number of bones in children's feet. Are there any other differences between their feet and adults'?**

A: Babies' feet almost always look flat—that is, there's no discernible arch—until they're two or three years old. That's due to the presence of a fat pad under the arch that largely disappears once the child begins to walk. With walking, a visible arch usually develops by about the age of four.

Other differences seen in children, such as "toeing in" or "toeing out"—in which the toes turn slightly inward or outward—also typically disappear by the time the child is seven or eight years old. Congenital problems that may require treatment are discussed in chapter 3.

Q: **I know I walk on them. But how much weight can the feet support?**

A: A lot. Foot care specialists say that your feet, acting as shock absorbers, protect the rest of your body from forces equal to one-and-one-half times your weight when you walk, two to three times your weight when you run and as much as five times your weight when you land after a jump.

Furthermore, even if you're not a marathoner, your feet do this mile after mile. According to the APMA, the average person takes 8,000 to 10,000 steps a day, which add up to several miles. So, the APMA says, an average day of walking brings a force equal to several hundred tons to bear on the feet. In a lifetime, your feet cover about 115,000 miles—enough to circle the globe four times.

Q: Who gets foot problems?

A: Just about anybody and everybody. The feet are arguably more subject to injury than any other part of your body. According to the APMA, 75 percent of Americans will experience foot problems of varying degrees of severity at one time or another in their lives. In a recent national survey of 1,000 adults, one out of 10 said their feet hurt "all the time." More than half of the respondents said they believed that foot pain is normal.

Some groups, however, clearly suffer more than others. Thanks to shoes with pointed toes, thin soles and spike heels, women are truly fashion victims: They have about four times as many foot problems as men do and account for a remarkable 90 percent of the surgeries for common foot problems. If they're obese, their plight is much worse. A 1996 study by Carol Frey, M.D., an orthopedic surgeon at the University of Southern California and director of the Orthopaedic Foot and Ankle Center, Orthopaedic Hospital, Los Angeles, found that overweight women are far more likely than their normal-weight counterparts to develop heel pain, **tendinitis** (painful inflammation of a tendon), fractures and sprains.

Other obvious candidates for foot problems are athletes, who subject their feet to enormous stress, and people in hazardous occupations; in any given year, about 120,000 job-related foot injuries occur, one-third of them toe injuries, according to the National Safety Council. In addition, people whose work requires them to stand for long periods, even if it's behind a delicatessen counter, are more susceptible to foot problems than those whose work does not require excessive standing.

Foot problems are a function of economics, too: People in lower socioeconomic classes have more problems than those in higher socioeconomic classes. And, as discussed in chapter 3, aging and certain chronic conditions, such as diabetes and arthritis, often lead to foot problems. In fact, these and other health problems are often reflected first in your feet.

Q: How do the feet reflect other health problems?

A: There are several systemic diseases that sometimes show up first in the feet. If you have a circulatory disorder, for example, the first warning sign could be a discolored patch of skin just above the anklebone—indicating that the area isn't getting enough oxygen. Swollen ankles can indicate kidney or bladder problems. Other conditions ultimately affect the feet. For instance, sciatica, in which there's pressure on the sciatic nerve—the long nerve stretching through the muscles of the thigh, leg and foot—can cause excruciating pain in the foot, as well as in the back and leg.

The humble toenail is often a leading indicator of systemic disease. Nails grow constantly, using a lot of energy relative to the small amount of tissue involved. That makes them exceptionally sensitive to outside influences. Healthy nails are pink and smooth. (Healthy nails are translucent; the pink appearance comes from the underlying nail bed.) If nails are discolored or deformed, that may be a sign of disease elsewhere in the body.

Q: What kinds of diseases show up in nails?

A: Redness beneath the rear of the nail could be a sign of impending heart failure. Poor circulation may be indicated by nails that are discolored, darkened, thick or brittle. Pitted or thick nails can be the result of psoriasis, a skin disorder marked by heavy scaling. People with iron deficiency anemia sometimes have "concave" nails, rounded inward instead of outward. Changes in the underlying bone can cause deformities of the nail plate.

Q: Are foot problems serious?

A: Most foot conditions are not serious and are easily treated. Sometimes, however, foot problems— particularly if they're ignored—can lead to permanent disability; in rare cases, they can be deadly.

Q: How can I tell whether a foot problem is serious enough to require treatment by a foot care specialist?

A: As with many other conditions, pain is a useful clue. Although, as we noted earlier in this chapter, many people believe that foot pain is normal, it *isn't* normal for pain to be so debilitating that it becomes difficult to walk barefoot or in reasonable shoes, let alone to run or participate in sports. If you continue to have pain after pursuing some of the do-it-yourself remedies described in chapter 2, you should seek professional care.

Another indication that a foot problem warrants treatment is infection, usually indicated by redness, swelling and, possibly, oozing. If it's a toenail that's infected—a condition described in chapter 2—you'll notice thickening, discoloration and possibly a foul smell.

Finally, if you have diabetes, as discussed in chapter 3, you should consult your health care practitioner at the first sign of any foot problem.

Q: Who treats foot problems?

A: A **podiatrist** is the primary specialist in foot care. Podiatric physicians (doctors of podiatric medicine, or D.P. M.'s) are not medical doctors or osteopaths, but they've trained for four years at an accredited college of podiatric medicine (there are only seven such colleges in the United States) and have probably done a hospital residency, as well. In most states, they're licensed to diagnose and treat—including surgically—conditions relating to the foot. After the podiatrist, the health care professional to whom people most often take their foot problems is probably the primary care physician—usually an internist or a family practitioner.

The medical doctor who specializes in foot and ankle care is an **orthopedist**, or orthopedic surgeon. In addition to medical school, orthopedists have completed at least five more years of training in surgical and nonsurgical treatment of the body's musculoskeletal system, with additional training in the care of the foot and ankle. While orthopedists are more likely to treat serious bone or joint problems caused by breaks or systemic conditions such as arthritis (see chapter 3), many orthopedists also take care of people with relatively minor foot problems.

Other specialists who may get involved in treating particular foot problems are dermatologists (when, for example, there's a stubborn skin infection of the feet) and **neurologists** (when foot problems are related to central nervous system disorders). Physical therapists may become involved in helping people relearn to walk after they've suffered foot or ankle damage or even in relieving the pain of acutely flat feet.

Q: Are there any foot care specialists who don't take a strictly medical approach?

A: Yes. Massage, acupuncture and acupressure are increasingly being used to treat certain foot problems, just as they're being adopted as therapies for other physical ailments. Massage therapists help work out sore

areas and muscles that have been overused. (See chapter 5 for a description of do-it-yourself foot massage.)

Acupuncturists use needles to stimulate various points
in the body to ease pain; acupressurists use their fingers
instead of needles to apply pressure to the same points.
While it's not clear how these techniques work, they're
sometimes used to treat painful and chronic conditions
of the foot when traditional therapies have failed. These
therapies are also becoming popular with athletes as a
means of relieving pain and speeding recovery from
ankle sprains and strains, tendinitis and fractures.

Acupuncture and acupressure can be performed by
licensed acupuncturists and other health care practitioners—including podiatrists—who have learned the
technique. However, if the condition for which you seek
therapy involves an infection or an untreated fracture,
you need to consult a podiatrist or other physician before trying these alternative therapies.

Q: Isn't something called **reflexology** used on feet?

A: Yes and no. Reflexology, which is a widely ac-
cepted form of alternative medicine that dates
back 5,000 years to ancient China, involves applying firm
but gentle pressure to a particular part of the body. Usually the pressure is applied to the soles of the feet, but
sometimes it's also applied to the ears or to the hands.
However, the object is to treat not the feet themselves
but other body parts, including organs, muscles and
bones, that reflexologists believe are directly linked to

certain spots on your feet. And if you have any foot
problems such as a damaged tendon or a recent fracture,
you should by all means *avoid* reflexology until you're
fully healed!

Some reflexologists believe that the pressure helps
because it breaks up toxins that settle in the feet as a
result of gravity and the constriction produced by wearing shoes all day. The medical establishment says that
reflexology works—*if* it works—simply because it's relaxing. Reflexologists are not medical doctors. Typically
they're physical therapists or masseurs with special
training and certification in this field.

Q: Do any other professionals look after the feet?

A: Actually, two other types of professionals—
orthotists and **pedorthists**—help ensure that
you're wearing the most appropriate, best-fitting shoes
for those problematic feet. A few fine lines exist between
the two categories. Orthotists, whose specialty has been
established longer, treat problems of the hip, spine and
hands, as well as of the feet. Pedorthists stop at the ankle.
Orthotists, however, limit their work to **orthotics**, or
orthoses—arch supports and other inserts that protect
the foot and improve the way it functions. Pedorthists not
only make orthoses but also can design, manufacture or
modify the shoe itself.

To find an orthotist or a pedorthist, ask your health
care practitioner for a referral or consult one of the
groups listed on pages 161-163. Some orthotists and

pedorthists are certified, although it's also possible to practice legally without certification.

In chapter 5, we discuss the types of devices that orthotists and pedorthists provide. Now let's go on to the problems for which—if self-treatment isn't enough—you might call on them and others for help!

2 COMMON FOOT PROBLEMS AND TREATMENTS

Q: What are the most common types of foot problems?

A: There are more than 300 different foot problems, but only about half a dozen of them are likely to bother most of us. According to the American Podiatric Medical Association (APMA), about 5 percent of Americans have problems with **corns** or **calluses** each year; 5 percent suffer from foot infections, including **athlete's foot**, other fungal infections and **plantar warts**; 5 percent have **ingrown toenails** or other toenail problems; and 6 percent have problems with foot injuries, **bunions**, **hammertoes** or **flat feet**.

Of course, since these problems aren't mutually exclusive, many of the same people may have a few foot problems simultaneously. And probably the most common foot woe, the **blister**, didn't even make the list.

Q: Why aren't blisters on the list, and what should I do if I get one?

A: Probably because they're usually too insignificant to come to podiatrists' attention. However, blisters—fluid-filled sacs that form between the top layers of the skin, usually as the result of the skin rubbing against shoes—can become problems if they're neglected.

If you get a blister, clean the skin. If it's not painful or swollen, leave the blister unopened. If it is painful or swollen, puncture it with a sterile instrument, keeping the top part in place to reduce the risk of infection. Apply a topical antibiotic cream (Bacitracin, Neosporin or Polysporin) and then cover the area with a bandage.

Q: What can I do to prevent blisters?

A: The likely answer—as you'll hear continually throughout this book—is to change to better-fitting footwear. If blisters are forming on the sides of your toes, your shoes may be too narrow; if they're forming on the tops of your toes or on the backs of your heels, your shoes may be too short.

In some cases, however, your feet themselves may be to blame. If you have bony toes or hammertoes, you might try putting a bandage or **moleskin** over sensitive areas or using foot powder to reduce friction. If your skin is soft, you can toughen it in blister-prone spots through the application of a flexible collodion product such as New Skin.

CORNS AND CALLUSES

Q: What is the difference between a corn and a callus?

A: Both involve excessive production of dead skin cells, which leads to thickened areas of the skin of the feet. And in both cases, the thickening is a protective reaction to persistent pressure or friction. But there the similarities end.

Corns are usually hard, yellowish circles of skin on the surface of the toes. (On African-American people, corns may be black instead.) They appear shiny and polished, and sometimes they develop a deep-seated, translucent center—a bit like a corn kernel—known as a **nucleation**, which enters the flesh in a cone-shaped point. Corns can also be soft and whitish, but soft corns—also known as kissing corns—are typically found on the webs between the fourth and fifth toes.

Hard or soft, most corns develop when toes rub against the shoe in which they're enclosed or against each other. Usually the culprit is an ill-fitting shoe, probably with a narrow **toe box** (the reinforced area in the shoe's tip; see appendix on page 159), and the usual victim is the little toe, which rotates outward because of too much motion in the front of the foot. But corns may also occur in proper-fitting shoes when toes are misshapen—for example, hammertoes, discussed later in this chapter, often develop corns.

Calluses, on the other hand (or foot), aren't limited to the feet—they can form on other areas of the body that are subjected to persistent pressure or friction, including the knees and the palms of the hands. On the foot, calluses typically form on the ball, the heel and the underside of the big toe.

Shoes—specifically shoes with high heels, generally defined as more than 2 inches—are to blame for most calluses. However, as with corns, the feet themselves may sometimes be to blame. Calluses may result if the metatarsal bones are too long or badly aligned, if the arch is excessively low or high (a condition, technically known as *pes cavus,* in which the arch doesn't flatten normally as the foot touches the ground), if the fat pad on the sole of the foot has atrophied (this typically happens with age), if the Achilles tendon is short or if the person walks with an abnormal gait or is obese. In addition, sometimes calluses form around warts caused by viral infections or around foreign bodies such as splinters.

Q: Are corns and calluses painful?

A: The larger they grow and the more they rub against your shoe, the more painful corns can become. Eventually they can break down, forming skin ulcers that lead to infection. Corns may also cause severe pain by rubbing against a **bursa**—one of the sacs of fluid that overlies and protects each joint in your body. If a corn develops on top of a bursa, as is often the case, the sac takes on more fluid to protect the bone. The result is **bursitis**, an inflamed and swollen bursal sac.

Calluses don't cause any pain when you're not putting weight on them; when you are, the sensation is often compared with the discomfort created by a pebble in one's shoe. The thicker the callus becomes, the more it irritates the soft, healthy skin around it. And if the callus has a nucleation, it can be particularly painful with pressure.

Q: How is a corn treated?

A: For temporary relief from the pain of bursitis, try soaking your feet in a warm solution of Epsom salts—available at any drugstore—and water. This will reduce the size of the bursal sac and take some pressure off the nerves nearby. If your corn is hard, you can peel off the dead skin by applying one of the several over-the-counter solutions (Dr. Scholl's Liquid Corn/Callus Remover or DuoFilm) or plasters (Clear Away One Step Corn Remover or Dr. Scholl's Corn Removers) containing salicylic acid.

Be careful not to overuse these products, as they can burn the skin. If the area is infected or if you have diabetes or poor circulation, don't use these products; consult your health care practitioner instead.

If the corn persists, you may want to have a podiatrist shave it down for you. However, the only way to ensure permanent relief is to wear shoes that fit properly and to use cushioned pads and insoles (see appendix on page 159). If you're getting corns because of a structural problem such as hammertoes, you may need surgery.

Q: What about treating a callus?

A: If it doesn't hurt, forget about it. But if you want to keep it from thickening further, you can try wearing shoes that have good arch support—typically inlays that provide extra support under the arch—and shock-absorbing rubber soles to reduce the stress on the area where the callus has formed. Alternatively, buy a callus pad or an insole that absorbs shearing forces inside the shoe. You can also keep a callus soft by soaking your foot every day or so, rubbing it gently with an abrasive brush or a pumice stone and then applying a moisturizing cream.

If the callus is painful, you can try the same salicylic acid products also marketed for corns. Or you can go to a podiatrist, who will use a surgical blade to pare down the callus and any nucleation it may have—a procedure you'd be advised not to try yourself. If the callus returns, the foot care specialist may prescribe orthotics—shoe inserts, discussed at length in chapter 5—to correct functional problems and provide protection, or he may surgically realign the metatarsals.

HAMMERTOES

Q: What is a hammertoe?

A: A hammertoe is a deformity involving a contracture of the toe, generally caused by a dropped metatarsal head—the knobby end of the metatarsal where it joins the phalanx—and a tightening of the tendons that control toe movements. Over time, the toe knuckle enlarges and pushes upward, putting the toe into a permanently flexed position. Hammertoes look like the small hammers inside the workings of a piano, hence the name. Usually hammertoes are the middle toes.

There are a couple of variations on the basic hammertoe. If the bent toe joint is the one near the tip, as opposed to the inside joint, the deformity is called a **mallet toe**. There's also a condition called **claw toes**, in which the middle toes curl under rather than flex.

Q: What causes hammertoes?

A: Although hammertoes are sometimes caused by foot injuries, they're usually hereditary. If you have a congenital foot problem, such as an arch that's so high that it pronates too little (see chapter 1) or a second (longest) toe that's especially long, you may be forcing your toes to bend into a hammertoe position. And you exacerbate the condition if your shoes are too short or if there's not a great deal of room in the toe boxes of your shoes.

Q: Are hammertoes serious?

A: Because of the way the toes buckle, hammertoes can become a big problem. As they become more rigid over time, the skin on the toes' knuckles becomes badly irritated from rubbing against your shoes. Calluses, corns and painful bursal sacs may form. To reduce pressure on their sore toes, people often alter their gait, placing undue stress on the rest of the body and sometimes causing hip and lower back pain.

Q: How are hammertoes treated?

A: A toe pad from the drugstore will treat mild hammertoes. Again, changes in footwear often will treat the problem. Wear shoes and stockings or socks with plenty of toe room.

If hammertoes are still a problem, minor surgery may be necessary to realign the toes. In a procedure called a **tenotomy**, performed under a local anesthetic, a podiatrist or an orthopedic surgeon lengthens the foot's tendons, allowing the hammertoes to uncurl and straighten. In addition, part of the bone may be removed to allow the toe to lie flat. Once you're back on your feet, you need to wear orthotics to raise the head of the metatarsal bone so that the hammertoe doesn't recur. (For more on orthotics, see chapter 5.)

BUNIONS

Q: What is a bunion?

A: A bunion is a bump that develops at the base of the big toe—a site called the first metatarso-phalangeal (MTP) joint. It's actually an enlargement of the bone and tissue around that joint. The medical term for bunion, *hallux valgus,* describes what is happening— *hallux* meaning the big toe, and *valgus* indicating that the deformity goes in a direction away from the midline of the body. In other words, the big toe begins to point toward the outside of the foot.

That's the start. As the toe increasingly angles outward, the bone just above it usually develops too much of an angle in the other direction. This condition is called *metatarsus primus varus—metatarsus primus* refer-ring to the first metatarsal, and *varus* signifying that the deformity goes in a direction toward the midline of the body. This creates a situation in which the first metatarsal and the big toe now form an angle, with the point stick-ing out at the inside edge of the ball of the foot.

The bunion that develops is actually a response to

the pressure from the shoe on the point of this angle. At first, the bump is made up of irritated, swollen tissue that is constantly caught between the shoe and the bone beneath the skin. As time goes on, the constant pressure may cause the bone to thicken, as well, creating an even larger bump to rub against the shoe. Ultimately the second toe may be pushed upward, so that it's constantly rubbing on the shoe. Bunions typically appear on both feet.

Q: What causes bunions?

A: A bunion is a form of arthritis, meaning that the bone beneath is degenerating, and like other forms of arthritis, it seems to run in families. People with flat feet are more likely to develop bunions than are people with normal arches. Bunions are far more common in women than in men. Possible explanations for the sex difference are foot shape and hormone levels. Women have a smaller, lighter bone structure, and because they have regular hormonal changes, the shape of their feet may change regularly due to fluid retention.

Once you have a predisposition to bunions, the condition is exacerbated by narrow-toed or high-heeled shoes, which can increase pressure in the toe box by 50 percent. Interestingly, bunions almost never occur in societies in which shoes aren't worn. Wide shoes with plenty of room for the toes will reduce the chance that you'll develop a bunion or, if you already have one, will help reduce the irritation.

Q: Are bunions painful?

A: Bunions cause plenty of pain from a multitude of sources. Particularly when you wear shoes, you'll have pain along the inside margin of the foot, just behind the big toe, as well as redness and swelling. You may have stiffness and discomfort in the joint between the big toe and the first metatarsal.

You may also develop a fluid-filled cyst or bursa over the bunion, and the skin over the bunion—which will initially become callused—may ultimately become ulcerated and potentially infected. The irritation caused by the overlapping of the first and second toes could lead to the formation of painful corns on the adjacent sides of those toes.

Q: Do bunions form only near the big toe?

A: Sometimes people develop a protuberance of bone at the outside of the foot behind the fifth (small) toe. This is known as a **bunionette**, or tailor's bunion, and it's caused by a variety of conditions, including heredity, faulty biomechanics (the way you walk) and trauma, to name a few. Like their big cousins, bunionettes often cause pain, making shoes very uncomfortable and sometimes even making walking difficult.

Q: What is the treatment for bunions?

A: For a start, take off your shoes and apply some ice to the area (three or four 15-minute applications of an ice pack per day) to help reduce the pain and inflammation. Or you can soak your feet in a solution of vinegar and warm water (about 1 cup of vinegar for every gallon of water). A **nonsteroidal anti-inflammatory drug (NSAID)**, such as ibuprofen, should also help.

Then step into a more accommodating pair of shoes, wide sandals or even shoes with a hole cut out for the bunion. If you catch the condition early, changing your narrow-toed, high-heeled shoes for a pair with wider toe boxes and lower heels may stop the bunion in its tracks. It will also significantly ease any pain you're feeling from pressure that your shoes are putting on the afflicted area. If a change of shoes isn't enough, try over-the-counter remedies such as bunion pads, which reduce pressure and rubbing from the shoe, or toe spacers, which attempt to splint the big toe and stop it from angling outward. Or try an orthotic shoe insert.

Q: What if self-treatment doesn't help?

A: If the bunion remains painful, you may want to consider surgery.

Decades ago, surgeons simply cut off the big toe, but you'll undoubtedly be relieved to hear that they've become more conservative. In fact, there are more than

100 different surgical approaches to bunions, many of them named for the orthopedic surgeons who developed the procedures—Keller, Lapidus, McBride and Mitchell, to name a few. X-rays will help your foot care specialist determine which procedure is most appropriate for you.

In the mildest of cases, surgery may be required only to reduce the bump by shaving it off and repairing some of the soft tissue in the big toe. But usually people require the fracture and realignment of the bones in the big toe so that the bunion does not grow back. In that event, the decision becomes whether to fracture and realign the first metatarsal, as well. The normal angle between the first and second metatarsals is 9 to 10 degrees. If the angle is 13 degrees or more, the metatarsal will probably need to be fractured and realigned.

Q: What happens in the operation?

A: There are two basic techniques used to cut and realign the first metatarsal. One is a **distal osteotomy**, in which the far end of the bone is cut and moved laterally, effectively reducing the angle between the first and second metatarsal bones. The bone is held in the desired position with a metal pin. Once the bone heals, the pin is removed.

In the other procedure, a **proximal osteotomy**, the first metatarsal is cut at the near end of the bone. The bone then is realigned and held in place with a metal pin until it heals. Again, this reduces the angle between the first and second metatarsal bones.

Then, to realign the big toe, the surgeon releases the tight structures on the lateral side (the outside) of the first MTP joint. These include the tight joint capsule and the tendon of the *adductor hallucis* muscle, which tends to pull the big toe inward. The toe is realigned, and the joint capsule on the medial side (the inside) of the big toe is tightened to keep the toe straight.

Q: **How long will it take to get back on my feet after bunion surgery?**

A: When the bones have to be fractured and re-aligned, it takes about eight weeks for the bones and soft tissues to heal.

INFECTIONS

Q: **What kinds of infections involve the feet?**

A: There are a number of infections involving the feet, including plantar warts, athlete's foot and fungal nail. (Fungal nail is discussed later in this chapter, under Toe and Toenail Problems.) Some are quite superficial and easily treated, while others often require professional care.

Q: What are plantar warts?

A: Warts, or **verrucae**, are benign tumors caused by common viral infections that the body hasn't been able to fight off. When they're on the soles of the feet, they're called plantar warts—because *plantar* refers to the soles of the feet. They're bumpy, spongy, sometimes thickened and scaly, and painful to slight pressure. They're often gray or brown, with a center that appears as one or more pinpoints of black.

However, not all sores on the soles of the feet are warts. Some, like calluses, are reactions to injury, hidden slivers or old puncture wounds. There are also certain cancers, including carcinomas and melanomas, that can sometimes be mistaken for warts. If you're uncertain whether you have a wart or another problem, see your health care practitioner.

Q: How do people get warts?

A: Generally the viruses that cause warts invade the sole of the foot through cuts and breaks in the skin. It's all too easy to pick up these viruses by walking barefoot on the tile floors of public locker rooms, showers and swimming pools (and on diving boards), on dirty pavements or on littered ground. For that reason, presumably, plantar warts are more common in older children and adolescents, but adults are not immune.

Q: How are plantar warts treated?

A: In many cases, warts go away by themselves within a year or so. However, if left untreated, they may grow to an inch or more in circumference and spread into clusters of several warts. Given that risk and the probability that the wart is uncomfortable if not outright painful, it makes sense to get rid of it.

Like corns and calluses, plantar warts can be treated with over-the-counter solutions (Dr. Scholl's Wart Remover Kit, DuoFilm Liquid Wart Remover or Wart-Off) or plasters (Clear Away Plantar Wart Remover or DuoFilm Patch System) containing salicylic acid, which helps slough off the dead skin. With self-treatment, small warts usually disappear in a week or two. Larger or more stubborn warts may take up to 12 weeks to heal completely.

If the wart persists, you may want to see a foot care specialist. He can get rid of warts in a number of ways, including injection with vitamin A, application of a caustic substance such as phenol or sulfuric acid or liquid nitrogen, surgical excision and laser therapy. Generally these procedures are performed under a local anesthetic.

Q: What is athlete's foot?

A: Athlete's foot, technically known as *tinea pedis,* is a skin disease caused by a fungus. (There are at least four fungi that cause athlete's foot.) Most often it occurs between the toes. You should suspect you have athlete's foot if your skin is dry, scaly, inflamed and itchy. It may also blister and crack. When blisters break, small, raw areas of tissue are exposed, causing pain and swelling. Itching and burning may increase as the infection spreads. However, if bacteria are also present, your feet will be wet and soggy instead.

Not all skin conditions are athlete's foot. Other conditions, such as extremely sweaty feet, reaction to dyes or adhesives in shoes, eczema and psoriasis (two disorders characterized by itchy, scaly skin), may mimic athlete's foot. To be absolutely sure it's a fungus, you could have the skin scraped and cultured. But most people go ahead and treat it without a firm diagnosis, and they're usually right.

Q: How is athlete's foot transmitted?

A: Often through contact between bare feet and the same tiled locker rooms, showers and swimming pools where you pick up warts—hence the name "athlete's foot." The warmth and dampness that characterize these places make them excellent breeding grounds for fungi. The fungus most commonly attacks the feet because shoes create a warm, dark, humid environment that encourages fungal growth. And while some feet are impervious, others succumb. The weaker your immune system, for instance, the greater your susceptibility.

Athlete's foot may spread to the soles of the feet and to the toenails. Because the fungus can last a long time, it can even spread to other parts of the body, notably the groin and the underarms, if you scratch your feet and then touch those areas; you can also pick it up from contact with contaminated bedsheets or clothing.

Q: How do I treat athlete's foot?

A: If you have a mild case, it should respond to an over-the-counter preparation that contains tolnaftate (Absorbine Jr., Desenex or Tinactin), clotrimazole (Lotrimin) or miconazole (also Absorbine Jr. or Lotrimin). Because it also has some antibacterial properties, miconazole is particularly useful in treating the wet, soggy type of athlete's foot.

Also bathe your feet frequently and dry them thoroughly, especially between the toes. Keep them dry by dusting them with cornstarch or another foot powder; you can put the same powder in your shoes and stockings. Whenever possible, expose your feet to light and air.

You may need to treat athlete's foot for four to six weeks, particularly if you have open wounds between your toes or on pressure areas, such as the balls of your feet. If your condition doesn't improve within two weeks, see your foot care specialist. He may prescribe an oral antifungal, such as griseofulvin (Fulvicin or Grisactin). However, griseofulvin is associated with side effects such as headaches, nausea and numbness, so it should be a last-ditch choice. If the infection is caused by bacteria, an oral antibiotic, such as penicillin, may be prescribed.

Q: Can I prevent athlete's foot?

A: You can certainly try, by practicing good foot hygiene. Steps you should take to deter fungal infections include washing your feet daily with soap and water; drying them carefully, especially between the toes; and changing shoes and socks regularly to decrease moisture. Wear light and airy shoes and socks that keep your feet dry; change the socks frequently if you perspire heavily. It's also helpful to apply a foot powder, such as talcum or cornstarch, daily to reduce perspiration. Finally, avoid walking barefoot. In locker rooms and around swimming pools, wear flip-flops or other shoes.

TOE AND TOENAIL PROBLEMS

Q: What other fungal infections affect the feet?

A: Another common infection is **onychomycosis**, or ringworm, a fungal infection of the bed underlying the surface of the nail. The fungus can also penetrate the nail itself, thriving off the layers of keratin, the nail's protein substance.

The first sign of a fungal nail is discoloration, but the condition is often so minor and painless that people ignore it for years. As the fungus spreads, however, the nail may become thicker, yellowish brown or darker in color and foul-smelling. Debris may collect beneath the nail plate, white marks will likely appear on the nail plate, and the infection may spread to other toenails, to the fingernails and even to the skin.

Q: Is a fungal nail serious?

A: If it gets out of control, it could impair your ability to walk. That's because it is frequently accompanied by thickening of the nail, which then cannot easily be trimmed and may cause pain when you are wearing shoes. This disease can frequently be accompanied by a secondary bacterial or yeast infection in or about the nail plate.

Q: How might I get it?

A: Once again, the likeliest places to contract a nail fungus are public locker rooms, showers and swimming pools—damp areas that nurture fungi and where people tend to walk around barefoot. If your nail bed has already been injured—by stubbing your toe or dropping something heavy on it, for example—it's more susceptible to all types of infections, including fungi.

You may also be more vulnerable if your feet perspire heavily or if you have a history of athlete's foot. And people who suffer from chronic conditions such as diabetes, circulatory problems or severely weakened immune systems are especially prone to fungal nails. The disease is very prevalent among older adults—20 to 30 percent have it, the studies say, though some podiatrists believe this figure is much higher.

Q: How is fungal nail treated?

A: That depends on the nature and severity of the infection, but a fungal nail can be hard to cure. In some cases, it can take a year or two to get it under control.

If the infection is still relatively mild, you can suppress it for months by cleansing the nail daily, filing off the white markings that appear on the surface of the nail and then applying an over-the-counter liquid antifungal agent. But the infection may still return, penetrating both the nail bed and the nail plate. In that case, you should consult your foot care specialist. He will culture the nail, determine the cause and prescribe either a topical or an oral antifungal, such as griseofulvin.

If that doesn't work, the specialist will perform a procedure called **debridement**, in which he'll temporarily remove the nail, scrape out the diseased nail matter and debris and apply a topical antifungal directly to the nail bed. If the condition is chronic and painful, permanent removal of the nail, as well as the soft tissue near the nail plate, may be necessary.

Q: If my toenail is removed, will it grow back?

A: If all or part of the nail is removed, it will eventually grow back—generally within six months to a year. Unfortunately, if the nail was deformed, it is likely to regrow deformed, as well. In such cases, your foot care specialist may decide to perform a procedure that partially or completely removes the nail so as to prevent regrowth. The procedure involves eliminating the **matrix**—the cells that grow the nail plate—either by surgical excision or, more often, by application of a chemical to the nail bed and matrix to destroy the growth cells. After such surgery, the toe takes six to eight weeks to heal completely.

Q: Are there ways to prevent fungal nails?

A: Yes, or at least to significantly reduce your chances of infection. Follow the regimen offered earlier in this chapter to avoid athlete's foot, keeping your feet clean, dry and protected from infection. Clip your toenails straight across to avoid developing ingrown toenails.

If you have a history of fungal nails, avoid wearing artificial nails and toenail polish. Both offer an ideal haven for fungi because they trap moisture underneath the surface of the toenail that would ordinarily evaporate through the porous structure of the nail. If you use a home pedicure kit, disinfect the tools before you use them.

Q: Besides fungal nails, what other toenail problems are there?

A: The most common is the ingrown toenail, a condition in which one or both corners or sides of the toenail curve and grow into the soft flesh of the toe. In most cases, it's the big toenail that becomes ingrown, but other toes can be affected. The result: irritation, redness, swelling, pain and sensitivity to any pressure—even the weight of bedsheets.

Usually an ingrown toenail is a minor problem, but if the area becomes infected, it can become major trouble. The infection may spread to the foot and the leg or into the bloodstream. You can lose the nail plate from infection or inflammation of the nail bed. Chronically ingrowing nails can cause deformity of the nail plate and the surrounding soft tissues. A small benign tumor called a **granuloma** can form along the nail margin.

Q: What causes ingrown nails?

A: Ingrown toenails typically develop when they're cut on a curve or kept too short, but there are several other causes. Sometimes toenails become ingrown under pressure, from narrow toe boxes or tight stockings; sometimes people who are bedridden develop ingrown toenails from tight bedsheets. Nails may also become ingrown as a result of repeated trauma to the feet, from running or other sports. Finally, people whose toes have a tendency to curl—either through heredity or as a by-product of a disease such as psoriatic arthritis, a condition described in chapter 3—can easily develop ingrown toenails.

Q: What's the treatment?

A: For immediate relief, soak your foot in warm salt water or a basin of soapy water. Dry your foot completely and then apply an antiseptic and a bandage to the area. If that doesn't help, buy an over-the-counter product (Dr. Scholl's Ingrown Toenail Reliever or Outgro) that contains tannic acid, which hardens the nail groove and shrinks the soft tissue, providing enough room for the nail to resume its normal position adjacent to soft tissue. To protect the toe while you're treating the ingrown nail, wear a soft foam toe cap.

If there's an oozing discharge, pain or severe inflammation, indicating infection, it may be a good idea to consult a podiatrist or other health care practitioner. He'll probably just trim the nail, but in some cases, surgery is warranted, either to drain the infection, to correct a chronically ingrown toenail or to completely remove a deformed toenail so it won't grow back. Even with oral antibiotics, the toe may take up to four weeks to heal.

Q: What can I do to prevent ingrown toenails?

A: Trim your toenails with clippers specially designed for the purpose. After the nails grow out beyond the soft tissue, they should be cut straight across so that they don't curve down and grow into the soft tissue. Allow adequate length for the nails to project beyond the skin at the toenail margins.

Q: Are there other toenail problems?

A: There's a host of toenail problems, most of them involving thickening, brittleness or discoloration. Many of these problems, which are discussed in chapters 3 and 4, particularly affect the elderly and athletes who subject their toes to repeated stress.

But here's one that's more likely to plague those women already afflicted with foot ailments caused by narrow-toed, high-heeled shoes: **paronychia**, an inflammation of the tissue adjacent to the nail—better known as the cuticle. Usually paronychia is caused by trauma or too much manipulation of the skin during a pedicure. The cuticle can easily become infected, and if the infection extends up the leg, things can get serious indeed. If you develop paronychia, treat it promptly by soaking your foot in a solution of iodine (Betadine) and warm water for 15 minutes, twice daily. Then dry your foot thoroughly and rub in an antibiotic cream.

A related condition is **onychia**, an inflammation of the nail-plate-growing matrix. Typically it affects the big toe and is caused by improper nail cutting, tight shoes or traumatic injury, such as a heavy object falling on the toe. The nail plate usually loosens and sometimes falls off, but the main object in treatment is to prevent or eliminate infection.

Q: Do the toes themselves develop any other problems?

A: Those infamous high-heeled shoes may also cause **neuromas**—swelling and inflammation of the nerves of the toes. The nerves become irritated and inflamed when they're compressed in a tight toe box or caught in the area between the metatarsal heads and the bases of the toes. The larger the nerves become, the easier they are to irritate. High-heeled shoes are the primary culprit, but trauma, arthritis or abnormal bone structure can also cause neuromas.

Neuromas can occur anywhere in the front part of the foot, but they're generally found between the third and fourth toes. One type of neuroma, called **Morton's neuroma**, occurs on the bottom of the foot between the toes, when a small nerve to a toe becomes pinched between the toe joints and the shoe. It's also possible to develop neuromas under a metatarsal head, particularly that of the first metatarsal.

Q: How do I know if I have a neuroma?

A: You'll feel pain, burning, a pins-and-needles tingling or numbness between the toes and in the ball of the foot. However, because these symptoms can sometimes indicate other conditions—such as **metatarsalgia** (painful inflammation of the metatarsal bones and their soft tissue sheaths, also caused by high-heeled shoes) and **peripheral neuropathy** (see chapter 3)—your foot care specialist may try to detect the neuroma with ultrasound.

Q: How is a neuroma treated?

A: You'll probably be able to clear up the condition by switching to low-heeled shoes with ample toe boxes—possibly with padding around the toes or metatarsal pads, described in chapter 5—and by taking oral anti-inflammatory drugs. If you continue to suffer from a neuroma, you may need surgery to release or remove the nerve.

SPRAINS, STRAINS AND BREAKS

Q: What kinds of foot injuries are common?

A: Among Americans over the age of 17, about
60 percent of all foot and ankle injuries are
sprains and strains of the ankle—specifically of the
ligaments, the tough, fibrous tissues that connect bones
to each other. A strain involves the overstretching of a
muscle, tendon or ligament, without any significant
tearing. In a sprain, there is actual tearing.

The ankle is particularly susceptible to such injuries
because the weight of your body is transmitted through
the anklebone downward to the other bones of the foot.
The typical ankle injury involves a sudden twist that
sprains the lateral ligaments (those on the outside of
the foot), tearing them from their attachment points.
Sometimes the medial ligaments (the inside group) are
also damaged.

Q: Who gets sprained ankles?

A: Just about anybody, from the basketball player
who lands badly on his foot to the couch potato
who steps in a pothole while crossing the street. You're
more likely to strain or sprain an ankle, however, if you're
overweight or pregnant (see chapter 3), if you wear high-
heeled shoes or if you've previously sprained that ankle.

Q: How is a sprained ankle treated?

A: Start immediately to use the following procedure, prescribed for any foot or ankle sprain, strain or **fracture**, or break in a bone:

- **Rest.** Keep off your feet as much as possible.

- **Ice.** Gently place an ice pack, or ice wrapped in a towel, on the injured area for 20 minutes every hour for the first 24 to 48 hours to keep the swelling down. The ice helps reduce swelling by constricting the blood flow.

- **Compression.** Also to reduce swelling, wrap the injured area in an elastic bandage, such as an Ace bandage, being careful not to pull it too tight.

- **Elevation.** Sit in a position such that you can elevate your foot above your waist, keeping blood away from the injured area to reduce swelling and pain.

To remember these steps, think "RICE"—rest, ice, compression and elevation.

Many people who sprain their ankles stop this routine prematurely because it often takes a couple of days for the swelling to develop. After several days of icing, you can soak your ankle in warm water and do exercises to increase the range of motion. If the pain and swelling continue and the ankle turns black and blue, you should have an x-ray taken to check for possible fractures. It can take six to eight weeks for a simple sprain to heal. A more severe sprain can require a cast and up to 12 weeks of immobilization.

Q: What parts of the foot are likely to fracture?

A: All the bones of the foot are subject to fracture, but the 14 bones in the toes get most of the breaks. Think of the times that you've stubbed your big toe on something in the dark! While not every painful run-in results in a broken bone, it happens so routinely that podiatrists advise turning on the light whenever you get up at night.

Fractures of the first toe and the fifth toe (which often gets fractured when you sprain an ankle) are extremely common. If it's your fifth toe, you're in luck. Often it can be treated by merely taping it to the adjacent toe, which acts as a splint. If you fracture your big toe, you can be in a cast for weeks.

Q: What other bones are susceptible to fractures?

A: The metatarsals, which are the bones in the forepart of your foot that attach to your toes, and the sesamoids, the two small bones that sit directly under the first metatarsal bone at the big toe joint, are the most susceptible to so-called **stress fractures**. The difference between a stress fracture and other breaks is that the bone is not displaced.

A stress fracture can result from sudden or repetitive stress. If a bone such as a metatarsal is overused, it will initially develop a small crack in the cortex—the outer shell—which over time progresses to a fracture of the bone. The second and third metatarsals are the bones most likely to develop stress fractures.

Q: How do stress fractures occur?

A: Often you have no specific recollection of what might have caused the fracture; you may simply develop a painful forefoot after some activity. Stress fractures are often precipitated by a sudden spurt in activity without proper conditioning—for example, a sedentary executive who takes to the tennis court, or a woman who, after spending months of her pregnancy in bed, begins walking again after she delivers. But stress fractures can also afflict superbly conditioned athletes, such as runners or basketball and volleyball players, all of whom often land suddenly on their feet.

You're also at increased risk of a stress fracture if your bones have lost density through aging, if you're putting unusual stress on a metatarsal because of a bunion or flat feet or if you're obese. And if you wear high heels, you're putting extra stress on the sesamoids. According to Glenn Copeland, D.P.M., author of *The Foot Book: Relief for Overused, Abused and Ailing Feet,* a woman wearing high-heeled shoes puts two-and-a-half times more weight on the sesamoids than when she walks barefoot.

Q: How would I know I had a stress fracture in one of these bones?

A: If it's in a metatarsal, you'd probably have sharp pain and tenderness directly above the break and significant swelling on the top of the foot. There's no point in having x-rays taken immediately, because they don't show the break for about four to six weeks. By that time, the fracture should be well on its way to mending.

A stress fracture in either of the two sesamoid bones is more problematic. It's harder to diagnose, partly because of the bones' proximity to the big toe joint, and it may never show up clearly on x-rays. It's also more painful because the bones lie within major tendons on the bottom of the foot. When you walk, these tendons pull on the sesamoids, creating more inflammation—a condition known as **sesamoiditis**—and pain and increasing the fracture.

Q: What should I do if I think I have a stress fracture?

A: RICE—rest, ice, compression and elevation (described in detail on page 53)—and anti-inflammatory medication are usually enough to help you get over a metatarsal stress fracture. Once the pain and swelling subside, you don't need to pamper your foot unduly. However, don't exercise during the recovery period, about eight to 12 weeks. And women shouldn't resume wearing high-heeled shoes during that time. Sometimes a foot care specialist may place a stiff insert, such as a leather or plastic insole, under the foot to hold the bone in place while it heals.

Sesamoid bone problems can take time to heal properly because there's poor blood supply and constant weight-bearing stress to that part of the foot. Often fractured sesamoids don't heal; the rough edges simply smooth off. If the pain persists, it may be necessary to remove the sesamoids surgically.

Q: Does the heel ever fracture?

A: Heel bones rarely break. Usually it takes a major trauma, such as a fall from a height of 10 feet or more, to make the heel fracture. Typically this type of injury occurs on the job, such as at a construction site. The heavier the individual, the greater the damage to the heel, which will fracture into more pieces.

Fractures that involve several breaks in the heel bone are repaired with a surgical procedure called open reduction internal fixation (ORIF). About half the time, however, people continue to have problems walking or working postoperatively and develop conditions such as arthritis. Many then have another surgical procedure, **arthrodesis**—fusion of the subtalar (below the ankle) joint. In fact, a group of researchers in Idaho recently reported that combining these two operations leads to more complete healing and less pain for the patient.

OTHER COMMON FOOT PROBLEMS

Q: **You've mentioned flat feet a couple of times—what exactly are they?**

A: Flat feet are simply feet with low arches—a condition created by an abnormal alignment of bones, an excessive elasticity of the ligaments or a muscle imbalance, or a combination of all three factors. Flat feet are usually not completely flat, although if the arches are sufficiently weak, they may eventually fall completely—a condition you've undoubtedly heard described as fallen arches.

Although flat feet tend to be inherited, arches can also fall as a result of obesity, prolonged foot strain from jobs that involve hours of standing or walking and—as usual—wearing narrow-toed, high-heeled shoes. As a result, more women than men have flat feet.

Q: **Isn't it bad to have low arches?**

A: That depends on just how low the arches are (or on how much you want to serve in the military, as flat feet have been used as grounds for denying enlistment). As discussed in chapter 1, arches are evaluated on the basis of their pronation—that is, the way they lower as you walk. If your arch falls flat on the ground, you have excessive pronation—and that's no good.

When arches pronate excessively, the muscles throughout the feet, legs and back try to compensate by tensing
and straining. Often this results in feelings of pain, such as
shinsplints (pain in the muscles of the lower leg), and
fatigue. Because weak arches take the brunt of the body's
weight during walking (instead of the balls of the feet
supporting most of the weight), people with flat feet
often complain of "tired feet."

There are numerous other consequences, as well.
People with fallen arches are more likely to develop
arthritis, bone **spurs** on the heel (discussed later in this
chapter), bunions, bursitis, calluses on the ball of the foot
and Morton's neuroma. Also, people who overpronate
badly tend to walk and run with their toes pointed
outward for stability, in a ducklike gait.

Q: Can flat feet be treated?

A: Yes. But they can't be cured. Flat feet will always
be flat. However, there are a lot of things you
can do to help the condition, from relieving pain with
moist, warm towels and gentle massage to using orthotic
devices that support the arch. Orthotics are discussed in
detail in chapter 5.

Q: So it's good to have a high arch?

A: No. It's good to have a *normal* arch. A high arch, or a **supinated** foot, is considered more elegant than a low one, but it's not necessarily better for you. In fact, flat feet—as long as they're not excessively pronated—may be better than high-arched feet because they can absorb the shock of walking over more surface area of the foot.

High arches don't absorb shock well. People with high arches often complain of pain in the soles of their feet and in their legs and backs. And often they develop severely deformed toes—hammertoed or clawed—with corns, painfully tight tendons and extensive calluses on the balls of their feet that make walking painful.

Q: Is there a treatment for high arches?

A: High arches, like fallen arches, can't be fixed. Often high arches are a result of problems of the nervous system—specifically, a disorder known as Charcot-Marie-Tooth disease. In most cases, orthotics provide considerable relief.

Q: How can I tell whether my arch is too low or too high?

A: Most likely, you'll know it when you see it—and you'll feel it, too, in aches and the related foot problems previously described in this section. But if you're unsure whether your arch is at fault, you should consult a podiatrist or an orthopedist. He'll ask you to walk, so he can observe your foot fall and your gait or use a computerized "gait analysis" that shows how you're distributing your weight.

Q: Apart from flat feet, are there other reasons that arches hurt?

A: One of the most common—and painful—causes of aching arches is **plantar fasciitis**, inflammation of the plantar fascia, the band of fibrous connective tissue that runs along the bottom of the foot and helps secure the arch. Athletes who run and jump a lot often develop this condition, but you can also get it from being obese or from otherwise putting too much stress on your arch—for example, by wearing shoes that are too narrow or even by standing on the rung of a ladder or step stool for a long time. The inflammation may be aggravated by shoes that lack appropriate support, especially for the arches.

With continued stress, the soft tissue fibers stretch or tear at various points along the length of the fascia, all the way to the heel bone. If the condition is ignored, it worsens. Bone spurs—spikelike calcium deposits, visible on x-rays, that measure up to half an inch long—form on the heel when small muscles associated with the fascia begin tugging hard on the heel bone. These spurs don't have nerve endings, so they're not intrinsically painful. But if they stress the plantar fascia, that can worsen pain that may already be excruciating. Also, because plantar fasciitis places undue stress on the Achilles tendon, people with this condition are at increased risk of developing Achilles tendinitis, a condition discussed later in this chapter.

Q: How can I treat a case of plantar fasciitis?

A: Get off your feet and take an NSAID, such as ibuprofen. However, resting provides only temporary relief. When you're up again, especially after a night's sleep, you may feel pain from the fascia band stretching and pulling on the heel or from the heel spur digging into the fascia. The heel pain may lessen or even disappear as you walk, but often it returns after prolonged rest. The reason is that the plantar fascia is trying to heal, and it tightens as it does so. One remedy is to wear a strap-on night splint, available at medical and surgical supply houses and at some drugstores, which keeps the plantar fascia stretched as it's healing.

Once you're on your feet, wear supportive shoes with stiff heel **counters** (the part of a shoe that wraps around the heel; see appendix on page 159) and good

arch support—for example, well-made running or walking shoes. Sometimes shoes with moderately high heels
will relieve pressure on the fascia.

If the problem persists, you'll need to see a foot
care specialist.

Q: How will a foot care specialist treat it?

A: He will probably prescribe a more powerful oral
anti-inflammatory or inject cortisone into the inflamed area. He may prescribe orthotics to relieve strain
on the plantar fascia, and he may administer physical
therapy, such as ultrasound or laser therapy. If the inflammation is severe, it may take three months or more of
therapy and rest before the plantar fascia fully heals.

If you still have pain, you may require plantar release
surgery—a procedure that involves cutting the plantar
fascia to allow it to reattach properly to the heel and
metatarsal bones. In rare cases, the heel spurs are also
excised. The recovery period lasts about two months,
during which you need to wear a cast and use crutches.

Q: Do bone spurs form only when there's plantar fasciitis?

A: No. They can also be caused by trauma; strain on
a ligament, tendon or muscle from activities such
as jogging or tennis; shoes with too much room in the
arch area; and obesity, particularly a rapid weight gain

that puts sudden pressure on the foot. And while heel
spurs are far more common, spurs can also form in the
front of the foot under a toenail plate, causing deformity
and pain. Some podiatrists consider the thickened bone
of a bunion to be a form of spur.

As we noted earlier, spurs cause pain by touching
other parts of the foot, such as the plantar fascia. If
they don't respond to conservative treatment, including
orthotics that fit your heel, anti-inflammatories and
weight loss, you may want to see a foot care specialist
about eliminating the spurs surgically. To avoid creating
scar tissue on the sole, the surgeon usually makes an
incision in the side of the foot to remove a heel spur.

Q: Is there anything else that causes heel pain?

A: Yes. Another common source of heel pain is
a spurlike condition known as **Haglund's
deformity**, or **pump bump**—so called because it's
typically caused by repeated rubbing against the rigid
counters of shoes such as high-heeled shoes. (Cowboy
boots, which are typically bought at least one size too
small, are also culprits.)

Haglund's deformity is an inflammation at the rear
of the foot, between the heel bone and the Achilles tendon. You are more likely to develop pump bump if your
arches are either very high or very low, because that increases the pressure and motion of the counter against
the heel. Pump bump isn't inevitably painful, but it may
become so if bursitis develops near the Achilles tendon.

In general, you can ease a pump bump with warm heat and low-heeled shoes. You can reduce irritation further by inserting heel pads in your shoes. If the bump—and severe pain—persist, you may need surgery to have it removed. This is similar to the heel spur surgery described on page 63.

Q: Earlier you mentioned Achilles tendinitis. What is it?

A: It's an inflammation of the Achilles tendon—the large tendon at the back of the lower leg that inserts into the back of the heel and attaches the heel bone to the muscle that gives it mobility. While other tendons in the foot can also become inflamed and rupture, the Achilles tendon is particularly vulnerable because it plays such a key role any time we walk, run or jump. For the same reason, tendinitis is particularly painful when it involves the Achilles tendon.

Achilles tendinitis occurs most often in dancers, runners and anyone who tries to push himself too fast, stretching the tendon beyond its limits to the point at which it begins to tear away from the heel bone. A woman who has been wearing high-heeled shoes for a long time and suddenly switches to sneakers, say, to exercise, may also develop this condition. Because her tendon has gradually shortened from regular use of high-heeled shoes, she may find it impossible to place her heel flat on the ground. If she then starts exercising, requiring the tendon to stretch, the tendon may begin to pull away from the calcaneus, or heel bone.

Q: How is Achilles tendinitis treated?

A: That depends on its severity. If the tendon is only mildly damaged, it may heal with the use of RICE—rest, ice, compression and elevation (described in detail on page 53).

You can also take an NSAID. If the problem continues, however, you'll need to consult a podiatrist or a medical doctor.

Q: What will a doctor do?

A: The doctor may put your foot in a flexible cast to eliminate some of the swelling and reduce movement, or he may put you on crutches to prevent your putting weight on the injured side. Your foot may be immobilized for up to eight weeks. (Most doctors will try to avoid injections of cortisone—a drug that causes adverse reactions, sometimes even rupture—into the Achilles tendon.)

If that does the trick, you'll need to spend an additional month doing exercises that stretch the tendon before you can resume normal activity. (That's also the prescription for prevention of Achilles tendinitis. Of course, another key preventive measure is to wear low-heeled shoes that don't shorten the tendon once it's healed.) If the tendon still hasn't healed, you may need to have it surgically reattached to the heel bone.

Q: What causes sweaty feet?

A: There are approximately 250,000 sweat glands in a pair of feet, and they excrete as much as half a pint of moisture each day, according to the APMA. Excessive perspiration, or **hyperhidrosis**, on the soles of the feet and between the toes is a common problem. In some cases, it is related to mental stress and nervousness, especially in adolescents and young adults. Systemic diseases such as anemia and hyperthyroidism may be associated with hyperhidrosis. If you wear socks that are made entirely of synthetic materials and shoes that are manufactured from manmade materials or that are tight-fitting, your feet will not dry properly, which can aggravate the problem.

Sweaty feet can cause rashes and eczema. Also, as explained below, your feet are more likely to smell if they sweat.

Q: Why do feet smell?

A: Foot odor, or **bromhidrosis**, is caused by decomposition of the bacteria that live on the skin. While it's normal, it's exacerbated by heavy perspiration, and people whose feet sweat a lot are more likely to have smelly feet. Further, if you eat foods that are particularly pungent or spicy, those smells are also filtered through your sweat. So to eliminate foot odor, you have to control sweating (and cut back on the garlic, among other things).

Q: How can I reduce sweating?

A: You can do a lot to reduce sweating by wearing appropriate footwear. A general rule is to wear thick, soft cotton or wool socks that absorb moisture. Avoid nylon and orlon (although some new synthetic blends are better at wicking moisture), and change your socks or stockings a few times a day if necessary. You should also wear shoes made of leather, not man-made materials, and give them a chance to dry out between wearings.

To prevent smelly feet, coat them with an antiperspirant or deodorant that contains aluminum chloride, such as Drysol, or use an absorbent foot powder or insole, such as Odor-Eaters. To kill odor-causing bacteria, soak your feet in a solution containing baking soda or a mild antibacterial detergent.

If sweating and odor are still a problem, see your doctor to get a prescription for a stronger medication to stop perspiration.

Q: Why do my feet get so cold?

A: Feet get cold because they're at the far end of your circulatory system and, along with your hands, are the last to receive your warm blood. While it's perfectly normal to have cold feet, if the skin temperature of your feet drops below 65°F (the normal range is 75°F to 90°F), you may have a problem with your circulatory system. If your feet and hands seem exceptionally cold, you should consult your doctor.

Q: What causes poor circulation?

A: Smoking is a major cause of poor circulation. The nicotine acts as a **vasoconstrictor**, making all your blood vessels—including the arterioles, the smaller-sized blood vessels in your feet—constrict and thus reducing their ability to carry blood. After you've smoked one cigarette, the blood flow to your feet may be reduced by as much as 50 percent, and it may not return to normal for a full hour.

Other vasoconstrictors include caffeine, amphetamines, some over-the-counter cold and allergy remedies that include ephedrine, and stress. (In some individuals, however, stress can have the opposite effect, increasing the flow of blood and causing the body to heat up.)

Q: Are there diseases that reduce circulation?

A: There are a few circulatory disorders, and these also keep your feet cold. They include **Raynaud's disease**, a relatively common and minor disorder that occurs primarily in younger women; and **Buerger's disease**, a syndrome that occurs mainly in men under the age of 40. In both disorders, the feet get very cold and even numb, but it's only Buerger's disease that involves the risk of gangrene, discussed in chapter 3. Both conditions are exacerbated by smoking.

And, as explained in chapter 3, poor circulation is a serious problem for people with diabetes. It's also more likely to affect people as they age.

Q: What can I do to keep my feet warm?

A: For a start, avoid the vasoconstrictors mentioned above, especially cigarettes. Don't wear constricting underpants or stockings, or open-toed sandals; do wear warm socks and other warm clothes. And exercise—that will improve your circulation and warm up your feet.

In the next chapter, we'll discuss measures that people with diabetes and elderly people can take to improve the health of their feet.

3 SPECIAL FOOT PROBLEMS AND TREATMENTS

Q: What are special foot problems?

A: In addition to corns, calluses and all the other garden-variety problems that are likely to trouble any of us bipeds, a host of foot problems often accompanies certain systemic and other conditions. These conditions include diabetes, arthritis, aging and pregnancy. In addition, people who have certain types of jobs are more likely to have special foot problems than the general population. And some foot problems are congenital—that is, people are born with them.

In this chapter, we discuss these special problems and how they may be treated. The foot problems that may occur during exercise and sports are addressed in chapter 4.

DIABETES-RELATED PROBLEMS

Q: First, what is diabetes?

A: Diabetes is a malfunction in the body's ability to convert carbohydrates—sweet and starchy foods, such as fruit, bread and vegetables—into energy to power the body. The medical name for this condition is diabetes mellitus. Diabetes is characterized by an abnormally high concentration of sugar in the bloodstream, so the key to controlling diabetes is to get blood sugar levels down to normal. Even with that, diabetes puts people at risk for a number of serious complications.

Q: What specific kinds of foot problems do people with diabetes have?

A: People with diabetes often develop a condition known as peripheral neuropathy: the gradual loss of nerve function in the extremities. Peripheral neuropathy mainly affects the feet, but it can also involve the ankles, legs and, at times, even the hands. It tends to be more severe in the foot than in the lower leg, and it seldom goes above the knee.

Q: How can I tell if I have peripheral neuropathy?

A: Peripheral neuropathy usually comes on slowly. You may not notice it at first because it is the absence or reduction of sensation. Some people say that they walk on what feels like "peg legs" because they have diminished feeling below the knees.

However, because the nerves are damaged, they sometimes create odd sensations. So instead of—or in addition to—numbness, you may feel occasional tingling, shooting pains, burning or muscle weakness in your feet and legs. These sensations can be mild or debilitating, causing severe pain and interfering with sleep and work. You may also have difficulty walking because you lose some control of leg movements.

Q: What causes peripheral neuropathy?

A: Precisely why this condition develops is unclear, but it's believed that something interferes with the body's nerve pathways so that nerve impulses are no longer transmitted properly. The culprit may be uncontrolled blood sugar levels (although many people whose blood sugar levels are kept within acceptable limits develop this complication), or it may be that the nerves are somehow damaged during the metabolic changes of diabetes.

Q: Does everyone with diabetes get peripheral neuropathy?

A: No. According to the American Orthopaedic Foot and Ankle Society (AOFAS), 40 percent of people with diabetes eventually develop neuropathy. The longer you have diabetes, the greater your risk of neuropathy.

On the other hand, the severity of the neuropathy does not necessarily correspond to the severity of the diabetes. Some people with mild diabetes can have severe neuropathy.

Q: Can foot care specialists and other health care practitioners test for neuropathy?

A: Yes. And anybody with diabetes should be screened yearly for neuropathy and related complications. Such tests may include an assessment of circulation, using an instrument known as the Doppler for measuring blood flow, and loss of protective sensation (LOPS). To test for LOPS, the health care practitioner holds a thin plastic wire buckled against the skin for one second and asks you if you feel it. Since LOPS may be patchy, she'll do this in several areas on the foot.

Q: Can peripheral neuropathy be treated?

A: Yes. It can't be cured, but you can take medication to deal with some of the symptoms. Until recently, health care practitioners mainly prescribed oral anti-inflammatories. However, a study by Robert Vander Griend, M.D., an orthopedic surgeon in Gainesville, Florida, found that mexiletine, a drug similar to the local anesthetic lidocaine, provides greater relief from pain and enables many people to return to their former levels of activity. Griend presented his findings at a recent meeting of AOFAS.

Q: Are people with diabetes the only ones who get peripheral neuropathy?

A: No. It can also be a side effect of some drugs, including certain types of chemotherapy for cancer. However, while the neuropathy is disabling, because most people on chemotherapy don't have the circulatory problems of people with diabetes, foot disease is not as problematic.

Q: So people with diabetes have other disorders that cause foot problems?

A: Yes. Diabetes can contribute to narrowing of the arteries, which decreases circulation in the upper and lower parts of the leg. Your skin and other tissues depend on good blood circulation for both oxygen and nutrition, so poor circulation can result in skin breakdown. This in turn causes minor cuts, bruises, burns and other injuries of the leg and foot to heal poorly. However, neuropathy, not circulation, is the main cause of most diabetic foot problems.

Q: It sounds uncomfortable, but is peripheral neuropathy actually serious?

A: Yes, partly because of the discomfort or pain but primarily because of the absence of feeling. If you have neuropathy, you can injure your feet without knowing it. While that may not sound serious, seemingly minor injuries—cuts, bruises, blisters, corns, calluses, ingrown toenails, even athlete's foot—can blossom into infections known as neuropathic ulcers, or open sores, if they're ignored. Diabetic foot diseases and disorders are the cause of 20 percent of hospitalizations for people with diabetes.

Q: How does a callus turn into an open sore?

A: Let's say the callus becomes extremely thick or dry and cracks. You're unaware that there's an opening on the sole of your foot, so it becomes inflamed or infected. The swelling compresses the blood vessels and arteries, which are already damaged or narrowed by your diabetic condition. These factors diminish the flow of blood to the irritated area, meaning fresh oxygen and infection-fighting blood cells have a more difficult time getting to the problem site. All this sets the stage for a serious infection.

Q: What should I do if I have diabetes and I develop an open sore on my foot?

A: First, given the potential danger for infection, consult your health care practitioner. If the sore is superficial, she'll probably treat it with topical antibiotic creams or ointments and tell you to change the dressing regularly. Open sores are usually allowed to gradually close on their own to prevent recurring infection.

She'll also have you keep your weight off that foot, especially if it's swollen. You might use a wheelchair, cane or crutches. Sometimes foot care specialists recommend a special walking cast, known as a **total contact cast**, which distributes your weight over the entire surface of the foot, decreasing the concentrated pressure that causes open sores. Total contact casts allow you to continue walking while you heal.

Q: How do I know if the sore is infected?

A: Warning signs of infection include an unexplained fever, too much sugar in the urine, or blood sugar that is difficult to control and requires a higher insulin dosage. You should call your health care practitioner if you have even a minor infection.

Q: How is the infection treated?

A: Usually with oral antibiotics. But the problem is that antibiotics, which are carried in the blood, can't efficiently reach the infected area of the foot in people with diabetes because their circulation is poor. Swelling caused by the infection further compresses the blood vessels and arteries.

An orthopedist can do superficial wound cleaning, or debridement, in her office, but if surgery is required to clean out infected or poorly healing tissues, it should be done in a hospital operating room. Vascular surgeons can sometimes surgically increase circulation to the foot and leg, helping persistent sores to heal.

Q: But isn't surgery risky for people with diabetes?

A: Actually, a study by William Costigan, M.D., an orthopedic surgeon at the University of Southern California in Los Angeles, found that the risk of surgery for certain people with diabetes has been overrated—but people with peripheral neuropathy or vascular disease still run a high risk of developing complications. If surgery can't be avoided, concluded Costigan, who presented his findings at a recent AOFAS meeting, people with diabetes and neuropathy or vascular disease should expect to spend more time postoperatively off their feet than would people who don't have diabetes, and their physicians should be especially diligent in caring for the surgical wounds.

Q: What if the infection can't be stopped?

A: The real danger with the combination of infection and reduced blood flow is **gangrene**. If blood flow were to be completely blocked, the cells served by the obstructed blood vessels would die. Once gangrene sets in, the only way to stop its spread is by amputating (removing) the dead tissue.

The first symptom of gangrene is coldness of the toes, foot or leg. Later the skin turns blue, then black. A very definite color line, called the line of demarcation, develops between the living and dead tissue. In people with diabetes, gangrene is typically "wet," and the tissue is moist.

At the first symptom of gangrene, you should immediately contact your doctor.

Q: Is amputation common among people with diabetes?

A: According to the American Podiatric Medical Association (APMA), people with diabetes have an estimated 67,000 "lower extremity" amputations each year—half of all non-trauma-associated amputations in the United States. According to a report in *Archives of Internal Medicine,* the lifetime risk of a "lower extremity" amputation is estimated at 5 to 15 percent for people with diabetes. That's 15 times the risk for people without diabetes.

For certain groups of people with diabetes, the risk is higher still. Presumably due to lack of adequate health

care early in the course of the disease, African Americans
with diabetes are twice as likely to have a lower extremity amputation than Caucasians with diabetes; Native
Americans are three to four times as likely.

Q: Is there any way to find out if a blood
vessel is about to become blocked?

A: Blockages in large vessels, such as those in the
legs, can be spotted with an x-ray called an angio-
gram. Bypass surgery may be performed to detour blood
around the blockage. In this surgery, a piece of a healthy
vein is "harvested" from another area of the body, such
as the thigh, and is attached at each end of the obstruc-
tion. The new vein directs blood to cells that had been
receiving an inadequate supply.

Q: Besides peripheral neuropathy, do people
with diabetes have other foot problems?

A: Yes. Another serious foot problem for people
with diabetes is a **Charcot foot** or a Charcot
joint, named after the French physician who first described this condition. It occurs in about one in 500 to
1,000 people with diabetes, but much more commonly in
those who also have neuropathy. A Charcot foot is more
common in people with diabetes whose circulation is
relatively good.

A Charcot foot may begin as a minor injury, such as a
twisted ankle. Because people with peripheral neuro-

pathy can't feel the pain that would normally indicate that something is amiss, the foot continues to degenerate. The small bones and joints in the foot become damaged or even broken. Then more bones become involved, until the structure and shape of the foot are severely and permanently changed. The Charcot process can include the collapse of the arch—the flat foot condition discussed in chapter 2.

Q: What are the symptoms of a Charcot foot?

A: Initially the foot and ankle may have unexplained swelling, redness and warmth. It's easy to mistake this for infection, and due to nerve damage from diabetes, most people who develop a Charcot foot do not feel the pain. In most cases, people develop this problem in only one foot at a time. Charcot joints may not show up on x-rays for as long as two months after the initial swelling.

Q: How is a Charcot foot treated?

A: If your doctor suspects that you have a Charcot foot on the basis of symptoms you are experiencing, the first thing she'll have you do is take your weight off that foot for three to six months. That may mean strict bed rest, crutches, braces or a contact cast because—due to peripheral neuropathy—you don't feel sufficient pain to let you know when you're putting weight on that foot. Most Charcot joints will heal this way, but sometimes they need surgery to remove bony prominences or to realign the bones to help restore the shape of the foot as much as possible.

While the swelling, warmth and redness will go away, your foot will never return to its normal shape. As a result, it's subjected to more pressure or friction from shoes and is therefore more likely to form sores or ulcers, which, in turn, can lead to infection, gangrene and even amputation. So while most people can return to a reasonably active life after being treated for a Charcot foot, they need to be especially vigilant in caring for their feet. And they may need to wear special braces or shoes for the rest of their lives.

Q: **Is there anything that people with diabetes can do to prevent all these foot problems?**

A: Plenty. Just consider this statement: According to the APMA, half of all diabetic foot amputations could have been prevented with early diagnosis and regular professional care.

For a start, get your blood sugar levels down to normal and maintain your general physical well-being. That includes regular exercise. However, don't exercise on your feet if you have a foot injury, because doing so might exacerbate a blister, bruise or cut, resulting in an ulcer or infection. Swimming is an alternative that gives a good aerobic workout, as long as you're careful to protect your feet with shower slippers or other footwear.

Then keep a close eye on your feet—particularly if

you have little or no feeling there. Check daily for corns or calluses that could become infected, reddened skin, sores, blisters, inflamed nails, bony prominences and changes in the shapes of your feet. Any injury, no matter how minor, deserves careful attention.

If you have trouble seeing the bottom of your foot, ask a friend or relative to inspect your feet for you. Alternatively, you can place a mirror against a wall near a chair in the bedroom or bathroom to inspect your feet. If you have poor vision, try using a magnifying glass.

Q: **What about daily foot care? Do people do anything different if they have diabetes?**

A: Yes. You need to take special precautions to ensure that your feet are clean and free of infection. Here are some measures:

- Wash your feet daily in lukewarm water, never above 95°F. You can't rely on your feet to warn you that the water is too hot, so test the water temperature with your elbow. Wash gently, using a soft cloth and mild soap. Dry thoroughly but gently between the toes.

- Use a moisturizing lotion daily, but not between the toes, where it could promote the development of a bacterial or fungal infection. Keep dry skin soft and pliable. Don't use hot water bottles, heating pads or heat lamps near your feet.

- Don't cross your legs when sitting. This reduces circulation in the legs.

- If you have good vision and can reach your toe-nails easily, trim them straight across with a nail clipper. Do not round the corners. Your best bet is to file the nails down frequently with a nail file or emery board. If you have difficulty doing this, you should have your nails trimmed by a podiatrist.

- Don't use chemical agents (such as the products described in chapter 2) to remove corns or calluses, and don't use inserts or pads without checking with your foot care specialist.

Q: I suppose footwear is important?

A: Absolutely. Poorly fitting shoes can give you blisters or ulcers in less than an hour. To prevent problems, here are some more guidelines to follow:

- Wear shoes with cushioned soles and uppers (see appendix on page 159) made of soft, breathable materials such as leather or canvas, not manmade materials. If you have peripheral neuropathy, consider wearing special "in-depth" or "extra-depth" shoes that can accommodate custom-molded insoles that help cushion your feet and prevent irritation. Avoid rigid plastic insoles. You should also consider shoes with a central upper section that laces or fastens so that you can adjust the fit as needed to maximize your circulation.

- Never go barefoot outside. Avoid sandals, thongs and open-toed shoes, too. Not only do they expose your foot, but they can also concentrate pressure between or on the toes, and the loose fit can allow the foot to shift and slide, leading to abrasions and ulcers.

- Before you put them on, always look inside your shoes for foreign objects. Make sure the shoes are in good repair and free of loose seams, loose heels and nails.

- When getting used to a new pair of shoes, it's a good idea to wear them for only short periods of time at first, in case they irritate in areas of which you're unaware. Also, in general, it's a good idea to change shoes during the day to relieve pressure areas.

- Wear cotton or wool socks, which provide the best padding—not synthetics. Make sure your socks are also in good condition, free of holes, wrinkles or lumpy stitching. Do not use socks or stockings with garters or elastic tops that can cut off your circulation.

Q: Will my insurance cover all this foot care?

A: Foot problems such as infections are usually covered. For routine care, you should check with your individual insurer. But if you have diabetes and are covered by Medicare or Medicaid—or by an insurer that follows the guidelines of the government agencies that administer Medicare and Medicaid, as many do—you should be covered.

According to the *Medicare Rules and Regulations Manual,* "Certain foot care procedures that are generally considered to be routine—e.g., cutting or removal of nails, calluses or corns—may pose a hazard when performed by a nonprofessional person on patients with a systemic condition that has resulted in severe circulatory problems or areas of desensitization in the legs or feet." In those circumstances, the manual concludes, professional care is covered. The manual states specifically that treatment of diabetic foot conditions, both medically and surgically, is covered by Medicare.

AGE-RELATED PROBLEMS

Q: **What special foot problems do older people have?**

A: Older people have a number of special foot problems and, while many of these include the common problems described in chapter 2, these problems tend to become more serious with age. According to the APMA, four out of five people over the age of 50 suffer from at least one significant foot problem—including diabetic foot problems, which often worsen as people age—and most require medical treatment for these problems by the time they reach 65.

Many of these problems are due to the physiological process of aging. Like the rest of the body, the foot is subject to the normal wear and tear of age and undergoes changes—from heel, literally, to toe—that cause discomfort and disability. As people age, their skin becomes more sensitive, making them more vulnerable to irritations and inflammations. They're more likely to develop problems such as plantar fasciitis (older men, particularly) and Achilles tendinitis (both discussed in chapter 2).

Other foot problems are the result of years of neglect or abuse: Women who have worn high-heeled shoes throughout their working lives, for example, may have to pay the price in retirement in the form of bunions. Still other problems arise because elderly people continue to neglect their feet—often by wearing shoes that don't fit properly or don't provide adequate support. Finally, other medical conditions, such as arthritis (discussed in the Arthritis section on page 94) and poor circulation, contribute to foot problems.

Q: Do the feet change as people age?

A: Yes. One of the most conspicuous changes is that the fat pads under the balls and heels of their feet tend to thin out, often to the point where these fat pads disappear. The result is increased pressure on the ball of the foot and on the heel bone—often leading to inflammation, pain, an increased risk of blisters and sores, and a burning sensation when they walk. (Because fat helps reduce friction, the less fat people have, the hotter their feet get with each step.) The pain is intensified because the nerve endings on the bottoms of the feet are

close to the surface of the skin. Standing or walking for a
long time, particularly on hard surfaces, as well as obesity,
make the situation worse.

Q: The fat pad won't come back, so is there any way to deal with the symptoms?

A: Rest will relieve the pressure on the feet; non-steroidal anti-inflammatories such as ibuprofen
or aspirin will relieve pain. Shoe inserts—such as insoles
or flexible plastic cups that fit around the heels—or
running shoes with a spongy underpad help support
the soles. If those don't help, a foot care specialist may
prescribe orthotics.

And it's not entirely true that the pad can't be re-
stored. Some foot care specialists try to recreate the fat
pad by injecting the area with collagen; the drawback is
that the collagen usually breaks down within a year, so it
must be reinjected regularly. Those who are continually
plagued by inflammation and burning and are willing to
put up with periodic injections may want to see a foot
care specialist for this treatment.

Q: How does the skin change?

A: As people age, their skin becomes drier—especially during the cold, dry winter months.
Skin gets particularly dry on the feet, partly because

they're under constant pressure, partly because they're the last area to receive circulating blood and partly because they're already covered in large areas with calluses (accumulations of dead and dry skin).

If callous areas such as the heel become extremely dry, they'll develop deep, fissurelike cracks. These can be quite uncomfortable and are also vulnerable to inflammation and infection. To make matters worse, older skin is also more sensitive and therefore more prone to irritations, inflammations and blisters.

Q: **What can be done about dry and sensitive skin?**

A: Calluses may be broken down with one of the over-the-counter salicylic acid preparations described in chapter 2. However, since many older people have problems with decreased circulation, this should be done only with the approval of a foot care specialist. Whether or not the calluses have been targeted for removal, the skin should be treated with a moisturizing cream two or three times daily. Moisturizing oils may also be added to bath water, although the drawback is that they may make the feet and bathtub very slippery.

Wearing socks made of natural fibers, such as wool or cotton, will help by absorbing perspiration, which can irritate sensitive feet.

Q: What are the most common nail problems in older feet?

A: With aging, toenails inevitably thicken, turn brittle, grow more slowly and become more susceptible to infection. For example, fungal nails—discussed in chapter 2—are common among older people. Systemic diseases, which are more common in the elderly, also leave their mark. For instance, people with chronic arthritis (discussed in the next section) may develop ridges in their nails.

This age-related thickening of the nails is called **onychauxis**. It may be caused by the reduced circulation that comes with age or by the small but repeated injuries that toenails suffer over the years. If the nail curves into a "ram's horn" shape, the condition is known as **onychogryposis**. Usually these conditions are painless, and cutting the nails keeps them under control. But since some older people may find this difficult, a podiatrist may need to grind the nail to make it thinner or file it down with a machine called a rotary burr drill.

Older people also tend to develop a condition called **onychorrhexis**, which is a longitudinal splitting of the nails—varying from a slight crack to a nail-deep split. Taking vitamins A and D orally sometimes helps treat this condition.

Q: Do the elderly have any particular problems with the arch?

A: Yes. One of the most common age-related foot disorders is a tear of the posterior tibial tendon (PTT), which runs down the inside of the leg, under the bump of the anklebone and forward into the foot. The PTT helps maintain the height of the arch and gives the foot its power to flex. But in older people, particularly those who are sedentary or overweight, it sometimes degenerates or ruptures. This may result in pain along the tendon, flat feet and instability while walking.

People who feel pain in this area should consult a foot care specialist. Otherwise the condition could lead to arthritis in the heel (discussed in the Arthritis section on page 94). The specialist may advise a person with arch pain to add a middle arch support, available from an orthotist, to her shoe, or to wear an ankle brace. A third, less common option is surgery to repair the tendon.

Q: If poor circulation is bad for the feet, as you've said, what can older people do?

A: As we noted previously in this chapter, people with poor circulation take longer to recover from foot problems or injuries. Since poor circulation often comes with age-related problems such as hypertension or heart disease, elderly people with these conditions need to take especially good care of their feet. If they take medication to lower blood pressure or alleviate

heart disease, that should improve their circulation—
and the health of their feet.

Q: **You said earlier that older people have foot problems because they wear shoes that don't fit properly or that don't provide adequate support. Is that really so common?**

A: Yes, according to a 1991 survey reported in *Pedoscope,* the journal of the Pedorthic Footwear Association (which represents professionals who modify shoes to help alleviate foot problems). The researchers surveyed 100 patients age 65 and older who visited their doctors' offices for problems other than foot disorders. Of these, more than two-thirds wore shoes that didn't fit them properly. Often the shoes were too small. People's feet tend to widen as they age, but few people buy larger shoes. The result: Of those surveyed, 75 percent complained of foot pain from bunions, hammertoes, corns, nails or the like.

While tight shoes can cause bunions and other problems, wearing shoes that don't provide support may be a bigger problem. A study reported at a recent AOFAS meeting found that about one-third of nursing home residents had only one pair of shoes—in most cases, slippers—and the majority of residents wore loafers, sandals and slippers. In the view of AOFAS, none of these shoes provides sufficient support. Less than 10 percent wore any type of shoe that provided significant support.

Q: Why is this a particular problem for the elderly? Shouldn't everyone wear shoes with good support?

A: Of course, everyone should wear shoes that fit properly and are supportive, but because older people generally are less stable on their feet, they need extra support from their shoes. Furthermore, older people are more likely to suffer breaks, such as ankle fractures, when they fall because so many of them have **osteoporosis**—a condition, prevalent in the elderly, in which bones lose density and strength and are more susceptible to fracture. And when the elderly suffer a fracture, the healing process is slower and the recovery generally more difficult.

Q: What kinds of shoes should the elderly wear?

A: AOFAS recommends that older people wear shoes that offer good support. That means shoes with a low, nonslippery heel, preferably rubber; a heel counter that's firm without being rigid; and adequate arch support. The upper part of the shoes should be made of a soft, flexible material—preferably leather, to reduce the possibility of skin irritation—to match the shape of the foot. And the shoe should be comparatively deep, to provide support all the way around. Most good running shoes fit this description.

In addition, socks or smooth-soled shoes or slippers should not be worn on stairs or waxed floors. In fact,

given the importance of support, socks aren't adequate
footwear for older people at all.

ARTHRITIS

Q: Does arthritis really affect the feet?

A: It certainly does. Arthritis is a painful inflammation and swelling of the cartilage (the soft tissue
between joint bones) and the synovium (lining) of the
joints; it's generally accompanied by an increase in the
fluid in the joints. It can occur in the back, neck, hips,
knees, shoulders or hands, but it also occurs in the feet
and ankles. In fact, almost half of people in their 60s and
70s have arthritis of one type or another in their feet or
ankles. The various types of arthritis that affect the feet
and ankle are discussed in this section.

The feet are more susceptible to arthritis than many
other parts of the body because each foot has 33 joints
that can potentially be afflicted, and these joints are
under continual stress from weight bearing.

Q: But what does arthritis do to feet?

A: Initially the feet become painful and stiff around
the affected joints. As the arthritis progresses, the

pain and swelling in the joints can affect the way you stand and walk. Ultimately the pain and swelling can become so severe that you can no longer walk even short distances. If left untreated, the feet and ankles may eventually become deformed.

Q: What types of arthritis affect the feet?

A: The most common type is osteoarthritis, also known as degenerative joint disease or "wear-and-tear" arthritis. Osteoarthritis usually comes on gradually, as aging breaks down the joint cartilage. Joints that are subjected to the hardest use or abuse are particularly likely to develop osteoarthritis. Ballet dancers often get osteoarthritis in their ankles at an earlier age than do most people who develop this disorder.

Osteoarthritis of the foot is also a problem for people who are obese. That is because the additional weight contributes to the deterioration of cartilage and the development of bone spurs—those spikelike calcium deposits discussed in chapter 2 that can form on the heel and toe.

Q: What about fractures or sprains of the foot or ankle? Do they increase the risk of arthritis later?

A: Definitely. A sudden and traumatic injury such as a broken bone, torn ligament or moderate ankle sprain can cause the injured joint to become arthritic in the future. While the risk is diminished if the joint receives proper medical care at the time of injury, it's still greater than it would be if no injury had occurred.

Q: **Does osteoarthritis typically involve the entire foot?**

A: It may involve the entire foot and ankle, or just a part. Presumably because the big toe carries so much weight and is subjected to greater abuse, degenerative arthritis is so common there that there's a term for the condition: *hallux rigidus*—stiffness or rigidity of the big toe. When the big toe is arthritic, it hurts as it pushes off the ground. If arthritis affects the rearfoot or midfoot joints, you feel pain when you put weight on your foot.

Q: **What other types of arthritis affect the feet?**

A: After osteoarthritis, probably the most common form of arthritis, and perhaps the most serious, is rheumatoid arthritis (RA), a chronic inflammatory condition that normally attacks the body's larger joints, such as the shoulders and hips, but often reaches the feet, as well. People who have had RA for at least 10 years almost always develop it in some part of their feet or ankles; sometimes the condition actually begins in the feet. No one knows for sure what causes RA, but it's widely believed to be an autoimmune disease, a disorder in which the body turns against itself and begins destroying its own cells and tissues.

Another type of arthritis that can affect the feet is ankylosing spondylitis, a condition that occurs primarily in relatively young men. Usually it starts around the "tailbone," causing lower back and hip pain and stiffness, but it can also involve the heels, making standing on hard surfaces uncomfortable. And a few types of arthritis occur in conjunction with other disorders or infections that also can involve the feet.

However, the arthritis most closely associated with the feet—specifically the big toe—is **gout**.

Q: What causes gout?

A: Gout, also known as gouty arthritis, is caused by a buildup in the joints—typically the big toe joints—of crystals of uric acid. This buildup is a normal by-product of a regular diet but occurs in greatest quantity in a rich diet that contains lots of red meat, creamy sauces and red wine or brandy. (However, **purines**—the protein compounds that can trigger gout—are also found in such foods as lentils and other beans.)

The crystals tend to settle in and inflame parts of the body at the far end of the circulatory system, so the big toe joint is a popular target. There, these microscopic crystals are attacked as foreign bodies by the white blood cells, exacerbating the inflammation. One or both big toes may be affected.

Q: You said some types of arthritis occur with other disorders. What are they?

A: There are several such forms of arthritis. For example, arthritis can develop in the joints of the ankles and toes in conjunction with inflammatory bowel disorders such as colitis (inflammation of the mucous membrane of the colon) and ileitis (inflammation of the ileum, a portion of the small intestine). Psoriasis, a common dermatological problem in which scaly plaques form on the scalp, elbows and knees, triggers arthritis in about 5 percent of people who have this skin condition. The foot is often affected—specifically, the last joints of the toes and the ankle—but usually only one side of the body is affected. The sexually transmitted disease gonorrhea, as well as pneumonia and staph infections (from staphylococci), can produce arthritis in the feet.

Reiter's syndrome is a group of arthritic conditions that may develop after an infection either in the bowel or in the urinary tract. (In the latter case, the infection causes urethritis, inflammation of the urethra, the canal through which urine passes as it leaves the body.) Reiter's syndrome typically combines urethritis, arthritis and conjunctivitis, or pinkeye, a common eye infection. When Reiter's syndrome involves the foot, it can attack the ankle joints, the small joints of the toes, the ligaments attached to the undersurface of the heel, and the Achilles tendon, or it may affect only one or two joints of the foot.

Q: How can an infection lead to arthritis?

A: If the bacteria get into a joint, they spread the infection. If the infection isn't caught early and antibacterial therapy started, it can cause severe, painful arthritis—inflammation in the joints. At that point, your doctor may treat it with indomethacin (Indocin) or another powerful nonsteroidal anti-inflammatory prescription drug.

Q: How do I know if I have arthritis of the foot—and which kind of arthritis it is?

A: You should suspect arthritis if you have any of the following symptoms in your feet:

- Swelling in one or more joints

- Recurring pain or tenderness in any joint

- Redness or heat in a joint

- Limited movement of a joint

- Early morning stiffness

These signs are particularly characteristic of osteo-arthritis. You also need to rule out other possible causes of inflammation in the feet, such as bursitis—an inflamed and swollen bursal sac under a corn (described under Corns and Calluses in chapter 2). In addition, different types of arthritis have specific symptoms.

Q: What are the specific symptoms of other arthritic conditions?

A: Arthritis that occurs in combination with other disorders has associated symptoms. If you have psoriatic arthritis, you'll also have dry, scaly skin; if you have Reiter's syndrome, you'll have red eyes or burning during urination. Any arthritis that develops from an infection elsewhere in the body first shows up as fever and chills, followed by swollen and painful joints. A doctor can confirm the diagnosis by examining a sample of fluid from the swollen joint under a microscope.

Gout probably has the most distinctive set of symptoms. It typically strikes suddenly and painfully, perhaps more so than any other form of arthritis. As a result, it's often misdiagnosed as an infection of the toe joint. But if you've just eaten one of those rich meals, and if you're a man (gout rarely occurs in women, and virtually never in premenopausal women), you should hobble to your doctor's office. Like bacterial infections, gout can be confirmed through microscopic examination of fluid from the big toe joint; in gout, the fluid contains long, needle-shaped crystals.

Q: How is arthritis in the foot or ankle treated?

A: Again, that depends on the type of arthritis. But in all cases, the objectives are twofold: to control the pain and inflammation and to prevent joint deformity.

There's no cure for either osteoarthritis or rheumatoid arthritis. Treatment for both typically begins with oral anti-inflammatories—notably aspirin. If that isn't sufficient, the doctor may prescribe injections of steroids to reduce the inflammation or recommend physical therapy, orthopedic shoe inserts or custom-made braces. Treatment of *hallux rigidus* typically calls for a shoe that's larger and stiffer, with an inflexible sole, to restrict the motion of the toe joint and thus prevent painful grinding of the joint surfaces. For rheumatoid arthritis, there's a wide array of second-line drugs—drugs that may be added if anti-inflammatories aren't working—that include gold injections. Researchers don't know how gold works, but it does relieve pain and inflammation for many people with RA.

The prognosis for many other kinds of arthritis is more hopeful. Oral antibiotics should kill a bacterial infection and cure the arthritis. If you have psoriasis or colitis, the best way to control or prevent arthritis is to keep those conditions under control. Gout responds well to the drug colchicine (ColBENEMID) and changes in diet.

Q: Is surgery ever used to treat arthritis of the foot?

A: Yes. Surgery is a last resort, but it may be necessary to reduce pain, improve function and slow the process of joint deterioration. It may involve cleaning the arthritic joint—trimming back synovial tissue, flushing particles of debris out of a joint capsule and smoothing rough cartilage. When possible, minimally invasive

surgery is performed using an **arthroscope**, a flexible
viewing tube with a diameter about equal to that of a
pencil, which provides the surgeon with an inside view
of the joint.

Sometimes part or all of a deformed bone is removed,
in a procedure called a resection, to help realign a joint
that is permanently and painfully dislocated by the inflammation and swelling associated with arthritis. Resection is
most frequently done in the feet when more conservative
measures don't help. Parts of the metatarsals—the long
bones that extend from the ankles to the toes—are most
likely to be removed; the bunion operations described
in chapter 2 are probably the most common resections
of the foot. A foot may be wider and flatter after this
surgery, but it's still possible to walk on it, often without
pain. In some cases, toes and ankles are rebuilt with
titanium implants.

Q: Is bone fusion ever used to treat arthritis?

A: Yes, primarily around the ankle. Bone fusion, or
arthrodesis, mentioned in chapter 2, may be used
to deal with the arthritis that often develops after surgery
to mend heel bones with multiple breaks. In that case,
people often have a fusion of the subtalar (below the
ankle) joint. Bone fusion is rarely performed on the
ankle joint itself.

In bone fusion, two or more bones in a diseased joint
are joined together to prevent the joint from moving.

The bones may be fastened in place with rods or screws to immobilize the joint while the bones grow together. Fusing a joint generally eliminates pain and can restore some function to a joint that had previously been useless, but, obviously, it also reduces joint mobility to zero. If it's done on an ankle, for instance, the gait will become noticeably stiff.

CONGENITAL PROBLEMS

Q: **What kinds of foot problems are people born with?**

A: First, let's note that few infants are born with foot problems. Whether because of bad shoes or bad luck (including heredity), foot problems usually take time to develop.

However, there are a few foot problems that babies have at birth. You've probably heard of most of them, although not in medically approved (or politically correct) language. These include, as mentioned in chapter 1, "toeing in" or pigeon toes—in which the toes turn inward slightly—and "toeing out"—in which the toes turn outward a bit. Other occasional birth defects include overlapping toes and **clubfoot**. All are discussed later in this chapter.

Q: What causes toeing in and toeing out?

A: It could be that the forefoot is turning in, or that a muscle in the legs has contracted too tightly. Toeing out may be caused by an Achilles tendon that's too tight. Granted, when they're first learning to walk, most babies turn their toes inward or outward a bit for stability. But the condition may become self-evident in the infant's first few months if, for example, she tends to exaggerate the toes-in or toes-out position when she sleeps. The diagnosis is confirmed if the condition persists after she's become an established walker.

Q: Can these conditions be corrected?

A: Yes. In fact, if the condition is fairly mild and if the child is still a baby, it may be enough simply to change her sleeping habits. Some pediatricians tell parents to have their babies sleep on their sides rather than on their stomachs or backs to keep them from toeing in or out. Sometimes parents are told to stretch the baby's forefoot at diapering time to stop toeing in.

Toeing out often self-corrects. If it fails to do so, the pediatrician may prescribe one of the "counter-rotational" devices that have been developed by orthopedic appliance manufacturers to deal with these conditions. While these are worn at all times, pediatricians say that children tolerate them well. If these devices don't work, it may be necessary to surgically lengthen the tight Achilles tendon that's causing the condition.

If toeing in persists, there are several treatments, depending on the cause of the problem. If the forefoot is turned in, it may be corrected by a counter-rotational device or a series of casts or, in older children, with surgery. If muscle contraction is the problem, most pediatricians put the child in a splint that he or she wears only at night.

Q: I can guess what overlapping toes are, but how are they treated?

A: Overlapping toes—in which, as you figured, a toe overlaps the one next to it—can usually be corrected if the toes are taped into the correct position continuously when the child is still under one year of age. Taping, if it's done early and consistently, can also help fix a toe that's not completely straight.

Q: What's clubfoot?

A: Clubfoot is a complicated malformation in which the foot somewhat resembles a club: The rearfoot is extremely flexed while the forefoot turns downward and inward. You should suspect that your baby has clubfoot if you see wrinkles underneath the anklebone at the outside of the foot, even when the foot isn't bearing any weight.

One out of every 1,000 newborn boys and twice as many girls have this condition, according to Daniel M. McGann, D.P.M., author of *The Doctor's Sore Foot Book.* However, in cases in which very early amniocentesis—a common test for genetic disorders in the fetus—was carried out on pregnant women, the incidence was much greater.

Q: **You mean that early amniocentesis can cause clubfoot?**

A: Yes, or a foot deformity similar to clubfoot. A Canadian study published in *The Lancet* in 1998 reported that early amniocentesis (performed 11 or 12 weeks into pregnancy, instead of at the usual 15 or 16 weeks) led to a large increase in the risk of a foot deformity. Of the women who had such early tests, 1.3 percent delivered babies with a deformed foot, compared with a normal rate of 0.1 percent. In half of the affected babies, both feet were misshapen.

The researchers speculate that early amniocentesis may damage babies' feet by causing a loss of too much of the amniotic fluid that normally cushions the fetus. As a result, the sac that encloses the fetus may tighten, squeezing and twisting the feet.

Q: **Can clubfoot be treated?**

A: Yes, and the sooner, the better. If it's only mild club- foot, it may be enough for a doctor to manipulate the foot to as correct a position as possible and hold it there with tape or a cast. Tape can be reapplied every few days or weeks for several weeks. If the condition doesn't improve, surgery is required—a complicated operation involving the release of the Achilles tendon and several joints. If it's performed in the first few months of the child's life, the surgery is nearly always successful.

OTHER CONDITIONS

Pregnancy

Q: How does pregnancy affect the feet?

A: In a number of ways. First, pregnant women carry around considerably more weight than women who aren't pregnant, and most of it is concentrated in the belly. So not only are their feet taking an unaccustomed amount of pounding, but their center of gravity is changing—putting additional stress on the ligaments in the feet. To maintain their balance, many pregnant women toe out slightly when they walk.

At the same time, the ligaments are being affected by hormonal changes. Pregnant women produce high levels of the hormones progesterone and relaxin, which relax the ligaments in the hips so that the birth canal can widen. The plantar fascia—the long ligament spanning

the distance from the heel bone to the metatarsals—
also relaxes, growing longer and losing its ability to control pronation, the rising and falling action of the arch
during walking. So at the same time that these women
are putting more weight on their feet, their arches are
less able to support it. It's not serious or even painful,
as long as the women adapt their footwear to their new
condition, as explained below.

Q: Whew! Any other changes?

A: A couple. Because the plantar fascia has elon-
gated, the foot actually grows longer and wider
during pregnancy. In addition, many women have severe
swelling in their ankles and feet in the final trimester.
This is because pregnant women are retaining excess
fluid, which obeys gravity by settling into the lower
limbs. So overall, the foot may increase by at least one
shoe size—in length *and* width.

Q: So pregnant women need to buy larger
shoes. Anything else?

A: Yes. A pregnant woman shouldn't just buy the
same high-heeled shoes in a larger size. If she
continues to wear high heels, her new center of gravity—
low and in front—will push her toes even more forcefully
down into a tight toe box. The result: sore toes and a
greater likelihood of stumbling and spraining one of

those relaxed ankle ligaments. Furthermore, because her feet have flattened out, a pregnant woman needs shoes that provide good arch support. The best solution is generally a good pair of running shoes.

Q: **But at least all these problems disappear with childbirth, right?**

A: Not so fast! It can take about six to nine months after childbirth for a woman's feet, ligaments included, to return to their normal shape. Particularly if she was bedridden during part of her pregnancy, she must be careful not to put too much stress on the plantar fascia immediately. And for many women, the change to a slightly larger shoe size will be permanent.

Occupational Factors

Q: What kinds of jobs create foot problems?

A: A great variety, from potentially hazardous trades, such as construction, to seemingly safe occupations, such as waiting tables. Some cases are fairly obscure, as in the chauffeur or bus driver who develops extremely thick calluses on his soles from hitting the brake and pressing on the accelerator pedals all day. Other jobs carry more obvious risks. For example, people who work with chemicals may develop **onycholysis**, a condition in which the nail plate begins separating from the nail bed after immersion in harsh chemicals. Athletes also tend to develop this condition as a result of repeated injury.

In fact, few of these conditions are unique to any one segment of the workforce. But they do tend to occur within some occupations more than others—hence the terms "policeman's heel" and "waiter's toe." (Metatarsal stress fractures, discussed in chapter 2, were once widely known as "march breaks" because new armed-forces recruits often developed them during the rigors of boot camp.) And of course, certain foot injuries tend to be job related.

Q: What is "policeman's heel"?

A: Technically this condition is known as **calcaneal bursitis**, an inflammation of a bursa just under the weight-bearing surfaces of the heel bone. It's generally caused by standing for long periods of time on unyielding surfaces such as concrete, as some police officers do—hence its name; however, it could probably equally be called "letter carrier's heel" or "assembly-line worker's heel."

It's easy to confuse calcaneal bursitis with a heel spur—the spikelike calcium deposit, described in chapter 2, that forms on heels. They're in the same spot, and they're both painful only when the individual is standing or walking—that is, putting pressure on the spot. Furthermore, if the bursitis worsens, it can lead to the formation of a spur. The diagnosis can be made by an x-ray.

Q: How is the bursitis treated?

A: You can treat it yourself by padding the heel of your shoe to ease the pressure and by applying heat to your heel to reduce the inflammation. Use a hot, wet cloth, heating pad or foot soak (two tablespoons of Epsom salts to a gallon of hot water) or a whirlpool bath. If the condition continues, you might have to have the bursa surgically removed.

Q: What is "waiter's toe"?

A: It's a chronic inflammation of the big toe, and wait staff tend to develop it by repeatedly kicking open the kitchen door of the restaurant when their hands are full of plates or trays. The inflammation can lead to an ingrown toenail and a corn beneath the nail. Treatments for these conditions are described in chapter 2.

Q: What can I do to prevent work-related foot problems?

A: Wear protective footwear and follow safe practices. According to the National Safety Council, only one out of four victims of job-related foot injury was wearing any type of safety shoe or boot when injured.

The APMA recommends certain types of footwear for specific hazards. Here's a partial list:

- To prevent injury from falling and rolling objects, cuts and punctures, wear steel-toed safety shoes, metatarsal guards, metal foot guards and puncture-proof inserts.

- For protection from chemicals, wear footwear made of rubber, vinyl or plastic, with synthetic stitching.

- For extreme cold, wear shoes or boots that insulate against moisture or oil and that can repel water (if this is a problem) and wear insulated socks.

- For extreme heat, wear overshoes or boots of fire-resistant materials with wooden soles.

- For electric current, wear shoes or boots with rubber soles and heels, no exposed metal parts and insulated steel toes.

- To prevent slips and skids on wet, oily surfaces, wear shoes with wooden soles or cleated, nonslip rubber or neoprene soles; nonskid sandals that slip over shoes; or strap-on cleats for icy surfaces.

So much for work. In the following chapter, we describe the appropriate footwear for people at play—participating in a variety of exercise and sports.

4 ACTIVE FEET: EXERCISE AND SPORTS

Q: Do people who engage in sports have special foot problems?

A: Yes and no. Although there are a few conditions that occur almost exclusively in people who exercise a lot or participate frequently in sports, most of the foot problems that afflict this group are the same that plague everyone. In fact, athletes—amateurs and professionals alike—share many of the common foot problems described in chapter 2, such as plantar fasciitis and Achilles tendinitis, with people who are obese or women who favor high-heeled, narrow-toed shoes.

At the same time, athletes do have a unique set of concerns. Their foot problems are not only more frequent but also more severe, partly because athletes often allow less time for recovery and thus aggravate the condition. That's why in this chapter we pay special attention to the specific foot disorders and injuries that athletes of all kinds—runners, slam-dunkers, tennis players, snow-

boarders and others—tend to develop and the measures
they can take to prevent or ameliorate foot problems.

WALKING

Q: **Let's start with walking. Is this a good exercise for my feet?**

A: It's an excellent exercise. As chapter 5 points
out, it provides fundamental health benefits without many of the risks of injury associated with running.
Your feet are required to absorb less shock when you
walk than when you run, for example, and you don't put
nearly as much stress on your arches. According to the
American Podiatric Medical Association (APMA), about
67 million Americans of all ages walk for exercise on a
regular basis—an activity also known as health walking
or fitness walking.

Q: **What kinds of problems might I develop if I walk for exercise?**

A: That depends largely on the condition you're in
when you begin a regular walking regimen. If
your feet are reasonably healthy and you wear appropriate walking shoes, such as those described on page 129,
you're not likely to develop anything more worrisome

than a blister. But if you already have common foot problems, such as bunions or hammertoes, those conditions could be exacerbated by walking for exercise. In those cases, you should consider consulting a foot care specialist before undertaking a regular walking program and consider buying orthotics for your walking shoes.

Q: But if I don't have any foot problems, can I just start walking?

A: As with any activity, it's best to start slowly. The APMA recommends beginning with five- or 10-minute walks, three to five times a week. Gradually work up to a brisk speed that will cover a mile in 15 minutes (or four miles per hour). To get significant benefits from walking, you must eventually be able to walk 20 minutes at a brisk pace without stopping. But, particularly if you're older, don't walk more than an hour at a time or seven times a week; give your body a rest to repair minor injuries.

Q: What type of surface is best for walking?

A: Smooth, level surfaces with some yield—a wood or rubber track, for example, rather than a concrete road—are better for everyone's feet. Especially if you've just started walking, avoid excessively steep hills and embanked roadways. Growing numbers of walkers, particularly older people, like to walk in malls in the early hours, when they don't have to step around swarms of shoppers. Not only is the surface ideal in most cases, but the atmosphere is climate-controlled.

RUNNING

Q: You mentioned that walking is less damaging to the feet than running. What might I have to worry about if I like to run?

A: Runners subject their feet to enormous demands. For example, during a run of 10 miles, the foot strikes the ground about 15,000 times, with a force equal to three to four times the runner's body weight. So, as you'd expect, most runners' foot and leg problems tend to be injuries from overuse, aggravated by excessive impact shock. These problems include stress fractures, Achilles tendinitis, heel spurs, plantar fasciitis, neuromas and shinsplints.

Blisters and toenail problems are also common. And of course, runners, like most athletes—and plenty of non-athletes—can easily develop athlete's foot from shared shower and changing-room areas.

Q: What special toenail problems do runners get?

A: In addition to the garden-variety problems discussed in chapter 2, runners and other athletes who put their feet to hard use sometimes develop **onychomadesis**, a condition in which, starting at the bottom of the toenail, the nail plate separates from the nail bed. This is usually caused by trauma, such as new running shoes that continually abrade the nails, in effect rubbing them off. Once the old nail has peeled away, a new nail often grows in, over the course of six months to a year.

Another common toenail problem for runners is the **subungual hematoma**—also known as "black-and-blue nail" or "tennis toe"—in which blood pools under the nail. Again, trauma is usually to blame: The toe is jammed hard against the roof of the shoe on every step and starts to bleed under the nail. To a degree, this comes with the territory, although it can often be prevented with the proper shoes, as discussed on page 129.

A subungual hematoma usually clears up by itself. While it's healing, you can get some relief from discomfort with cool compresses or ice. If the condition persists or is quite painful, you should consult a foot care specialist, who may drain the blood by drilling a small hole in the nail.

Q: Is it true that running on concrete rather than, say, grass, is harder on the feet?

A: It's true that because concrete doesn't absorb shocks as grass or a dirt road does, a runner's legs, feet and back can take a greater pounding. But each type of surface can cause different types of foot problems.

Grass surfaces are often irregular, so runners can more easily sprain their ankles. Similarly, running on a sloping or banked surface may cause the foot to rotate excessively and may place additional stress on the tendons and ligaments of the leg and foot. (However, the good news is that because runners don't take the sharp diagonal cuts used in contact sports, described on page 120, they tend to be relatively free of ankle sprains.) Uphill running places a strain on the Achilles tendon and muscles of the lower back; downhill running places a lot of pressure on the heel.

The ideal running surface is relatively smooth, level and shock-absorbent—probably like the wood or rubber track at your gym.

Q: What about foot cramps?

A: Runners, as well as other athletes, sometimes develop cramping—a sudden and sustained spasm of a muscle—in the calf muscles or feet. No one knows for sure what causes this cramping, but one theory is that an imbalance of electrolytes and fluid, often the result of the loss of fluids through heavy sweating, may be responsible. Sometimes athletes also get cramping at night, due to muscle tightness or overuse that has led to a buildup of lactic acid in the muscle. (Lactic acid is the end product of muscle contraction, a by-product of metabolism.) To decrease its buildup, stretch after you exercise to improve your circulation.

CONTACT AND OTHER TEAM SPORTS

Q: What are the foot problems for athletes in contact sports?

A: While runners typically suffer foot problems from overuse, people who play contact sports such as football and soccer are far more likely to suffer impact or trauma injuries from hard tackling, pileups and quick changes in direction. Their feet get stepped on, kicked, jammed, twisted and cut. Their ankles get sprained and fractured, muscles get pulled, and tendons are ruptured.

The typical contact sport injury is a sprained or torn lateral ligament—a ligament on the outside of the foot— that occurs when the player's foot remains stationary while his body rotates. But players also get fractures— both stress fractures, in which the bone is not displaced, and complete fractures, in which it is—and something called "turf toe."

Q: What's turf toe?

A: It's a painful hyperextension of the big toe, and its name comes from the artificial turf that's considered largely to blame for the condition. Because artificial turf is harder and less yielding than grass, it allows players to pick up speed. Turf toe typically develops when a player stubs his toe or changes directions while running at breakneck speed or gets hit after planting his forefoot in the turf and raising his heel.

To make matters worse, many football players have adopted lighter-weight shoes to take advantage of the greater speed afforded by artificial turf. These shoes are more flexible, but they increase the stress directly on the toe joints, leading to still more sprains. Athletes playing on artificial turf have to modify the way they run and change direction, and they often tape their feet and ankles for added stability.

Q: What does slam-dunking do to feet?

A: Slam-dunking and other high-flying basketball feats exert tremendous pressure on the feet and ankles. In basketball, most acute foot and ankle injuries—that is, injuries from sudden and forceful blows—are caused by landing too hard on one part of the foot or twisting while falling. The most common such injuries include ankle sprains, torn ligaments, muscle pulls, tendon ruptures and fractures. Basketball players also have multiple overuse injuries and disorders: stress fractures, plantar fasciitis, shinsplints, Achilles tendinitis, sesamoiditis and blisters.

Q: **Does the playing surface make a difference?**

A: Yes, just as it does with football and running. Indoor wood courts offer the most shock absorption and are therefore considered the safest courts. Asphalt or concrete courts are the hardest and most dangerous for players' feet.

Q: **Apart from those you've described, do football, basketball and soccer players get other foot or ankle injuries?**

A: Yes. It's not uncommon for basketball, football, soccer and volleyball players to develop a condition called **osteochondritis dissecans (OCD)**, which is a deep bruise of the joint involving the cartilage surface and underlying bone. While it can affect a number of joints, OCD typically develops in the talus bone (the saddle-shaped bone at the base of the ankle) after an ankle sprain or other injury.

OCD is painful and can be debilitating if the bruise doesn't heal. In that event, the cartilage and bone that have been damaged by the injury will loosen and rub against exposed bone, causing immense pain. It's also painful to walk and run on the unprotected bone without its usual shock-absorbing cushion of cartilage.

Q: Can OCD be treated?

A: Yes, with surgery. In the past, the talus was repaired with synthetic materials or bone and cartilage from cadavers. Recently, however, surgeons have begun treating OCD with **mosaicplasty**, a technique that had previously been used to repair knee joints. The procedure involves transplanting small amounts of cartilage and bone from the non-weight-bearing parts of the knee to the damaged talus.

A recent study in *Foot and Ankle International,* the journal of the American Orthopaedic Foot and Ankle Society (AOFAS), reported excellent results with this technique. The principal researcher, Gary Kish, M.D., a Portsmouth, New Hampshire, orthopedic surgeon who is team physician for the University of New Hampshire football program, reported that using the person's own tissue reduced the risk that the patient would either develop an infection or reject the transplanted material.

Q: What about tamer sports such as baseball? Are they associated with foot problems?

A: Here's a list of a few of those sports and the foot disorders to which players are susceptible. While these sports aren't as problematic for the feet as, for example, basketball, they do have perils of their own.

- *Baseball.* Sliding into home plate may be the highlight of a game, but it can also be perilous for the feet, causing sprains and even fractures of the lower leg and foot. Certain positions have specific hazards: Catchers can develop plantar fasciitis and heel spurs from squatting behind home plate; pitchers can develop other "overuse" problems from the repetitive motion of stepping back and forth on the pitching mound. For all players, common foot problems include contusions, or bruises, from a baseball accidentally hitting a player's foot or ankle; sprains and fractures, from running or pivoting to make a play; shinsplints, from running; and Achilles tendinitis, from the stop-and-start nature of baseball—the long waits between sprints.

- *Tennis and other racket sports* (badminton, paddle tennis, racquetball or squash). As noted earlier, the subungual hematoma is also known as tennis toe and often occurs when the player's toe is jammed hard against the roof of the shoe. Other common problems are ankle sprains, stress fractures and plantar fasciitis. Injuries are less likely to occur on clay courts and the new crushed stone "fast-dry" courts, which are soft and let players slide on the surface. Players run the greater risk on outdoor courts that are surfaced with asphalt or concrete, and indoor courts with carpeting, none of which allows for sliding.

- *Golf.* While even the most inept golfer would be hard put to injure his feet in a game, the positioning and weight-bearing of the feet play an important role in a golf swing—hence the importance of healthy feet. Wearing inappropriate or ill-fitting shoes for 18 holes can bring on blisters, neuromas and other foot pain—not unlike the problems we've attributed to women's high-heeled, narrow-toed shoes in earlier chapters.

- **In-line skating.** Most in-line skating injuries involve the wrist, not the foot. A study commissioned by Rollerblade, a leading manufacturer, and conducted by the University of Massachusetts Exercise Science Department found that in-line skating provided an aerobic workout comparable to running, with only half the impact shock on the lower leg. However, skates that don't fit properly—where, for example, there's too much pressure on the top of the foot—can cause blisters, neuromas and other common foot problems.

WINTER SPORTS

Q: Do snowboarders have special foot problems?

A: Yes. In fact, they have their own condition, called snowboarder's fracture—a hard-to-detect fracture of the talus bone. According to a study published in a recent issue of the *American Journal of Sports Medicine,* 15 percent of all ankle injuries sustained by snowboarders are snowboarder's fractures. The author of the study, Douglas Kirkpatrick, M.D., an orthopedic surgeon in Queensbury, New York, says these fractures occur in snowboarders because the flexibility of their boots, compared with skiers', and the attachment of both feet to the board lead to more up-and-down movement and twisting.

Because the talus bone can be very difficult to see with x-rays, these fractures are often misdiagnosed as sprains. If neglected, however, they can lead to a loss of motion below the talus bone as well as the development of arthritis in the subtalar joint (the joint formed by the ankle and the heel bone) within a year or two.

If your ankle continues to hurt for days after you've been snowboarding and x-rays don't shed any light, ask your doctor about having a CT (or CAT) scan—a detailed, three-dimensional image similar to an x-ray—which would clearly show the fracture.

Q: **What about other winter sports? Aren't they all pretty hard on the feet?**

A: You probably associate skiing, and possibly ice skating, with broken ankles, but such risks are considerably reduced if your ski boots or skates are designed well and fit properly. But there are other potential problems. Just as with shoes, ski boots or skates that are too narrow can cause neuromas or aggravate preexisting bone problems, such as bunions and hammertoes. Pressure in the toe box can cause a subungual hematoma, and friction in winter sports footwear often causes blisters.

Cross-country skiing is more like running than like downhill skiing: The shoe is softer, like an athletic or running shoe, and the potential injuries are similar. The constant up-and-down motion of the heel—the shoe is bound to the ski only at the toe—can result in Achilles tendinitis, plantar fasciitis and blisters.

And when it comes to feet, athletes who engage in these activities should never overlook the danger of **frostbite**.

Q: What exactly is frostbite?

A: Frostbite is the freezing of tissues caused by their overexposure to extreme cold. To maintain a normal temperature for the vital organs in cold weather, the body reduces the flow of blood to the skin surface and extremities—the feet and hands. Minor frostbite may cause only blanching of the skin; severe frostbite may result in the loss of fingers and toes.

With feet, the particular danger is that you can't see the skin color change under a boot or skate. However, if your toes are extremely cold for a prolonged period or you feel burning or numbness, you may be at risk for frostbite. Immobility, wet clothing, lack of proper clothing and exhaustion increase your risk.

Q: How do I treat frostbitten toes?

A: First, let's dispel one misconception about frostbite: You *don't* improve things by rubbing the affected area with ice or snow. That seems to provide warmth, but it only worsens the situation because the ice crystals may lacerate, or tear, the cells. You should also avoid alcohol (which may make you feel warmer but, in fact, increases the loss of body heat) and nicotine (which, as noted in chapter 2, narrows the blood vessels). If you're using a nicotine gum or patch to help you quit smoking, you should avoid them when you're exposed to extreme cold.

Here's what you *should do* to treat frostbite:

- Promptly immerse the frostbitten foot in warm, not hot, water (104°F to 108°F).

- Rewarm the water and immerse the foot until a flush returns to the tips of the toes. This usually takes about 20 to 30 minutes. (Avoid dry heat because you could accidentally burn the skin.)

- If possible, soak the foot for about 20 minutes in a whirlpool bath once or twice daily until the affected area recovers its normal color and sensation.

If you've ever been frostbitten, even if you recover fully, you must be extra careful not to expose yourself again to extreme cold for hours at a time.

Q: **Why do I have to be more careful?**

A: In anyone who's been frostbitten, some of the tiny blood vessels at the end of the toes are permanently damaged, reducing circulation to those areas. In cold weather, the blood vessels naturally constrict, or narrow, further reducing the supply of blood to your toes. That makes you more susceptible to another case of frostbite in the same place. Particularly if you're at risk, you should consider measures such as the battery-powered heated ski boots that are now available. Alternatively, and more economically, you could try disposable boot warmers—inserts that heat up chemically when their paper backing is removed.

ATHLETIC SHOES

Q: How do I know which type of shoe is best for my particular sport?

A: With the proliferation of athletic shoes for runners, walkers, cross-trainers and just about everybody else, it's hard to know what's best for any one sport. You don't necessarily need to change shoes every time you change sports. Generally, according to AOFAS, you should wear sport-specific shoes for sports you play more than three times a week.

Q: OK, let's say I run or walk vigorously that often. What should I wear?

A: Keep in mind that your specific shoe choice should be influenced by your weight (heavier people need more shock absorption), your foot structure, the intensity with which you participate in your sport and the surface on which you do it. Here are some guidelines for the most foot-intensive activities:

- *Running.* Unlike shoes for tennis and many other sports, running shoes are designed to move you in only one direction—straight ahead. Soles curve up in front and back—a "rocker bottom" that helps to smoothly shift weight from the heel to the toes, while decreasing the forces across the foot. The heel is slightly elevated, with a beveled edge for stability. The uppers are nylon, with suede, leather or pigskin at the stress points. Running shoes should provide maximum overall shock absorption for the feet. They should also be able to bend fully at the ball of the foot area. Running shoes fit properly if the heel is snug and does not slide and if there is a thumb's width between the longest toe and the tip of the toe box. You should be able to wiggle your toes.

- *Walking.* Walking shoes tend to be somewhat lighter than running shoes, with slightly less cushioning. However, there should be good shock absorption in the heel of the shoe and especially under the ball of the foot. Like running shoes, shoes for walking should have a rocker bottom and a slightly elevated heel. Walking shoes have more rigidity in the front, so you can roll off your toes rather than bend through them as you do with running shoes. Uppers are nylon mesh or leather.

- *Aerobics.* Because vigorous aerobics involves quick lateral movements, jumping and leaping, all of which can cause stress fractures, you need exercise-specific shoes, according to the American Aerobics Association International. Running and walking shoes lack the necessary lateral stability and lift the heel too high. Aerobics shoes should have ample cushioning to lessen impact, particularly in the sole beneath the ball of the foot, where the greatest stress occurs. Shoes also need an arch designed to support frequent side-to-side motion and a thick upper to provide forefoot stability. Aerobic shoes are made of soft leather, canvas or nylon. They should be tied securely—tightly around the arch, but loosely enough so that you can spread your toes.

- *Cross-training.* Shoes for cross-trainers should provide adequate stability, shock absorption and flexibility for a variety of sports—running, tennis, aerobics, bicycling. Compared with running shoes, cross-trainers may have more cushioning for forefoot shock absorption, less cushioning for the rearfoot.

Q: What about recent innovations like air pockets and pumps?

A: Most of these modifications have been introduced by manufacturers to increase shock absorption. They include the Nike Air line, which has air pockets at the bottom of the shoe from the rearfoot to the midfoot. Then there are Tiger Gels (manufactured by Tiger), which use a gel instead of air in the pockets, and a HydroFlow line (manufactured by Brooks) with water instead of air or gel.

In addition, Reebok has a line of high-tops that come with an air bladder that can be pumped up or released to mold to the shape of the foot, for added ankle support.

Q: Are these gimmicks, or do they actually make a difference?

A: That's debatable. While Glenn Copeland, D.P.M., author of *The Foot Book,* doesn't make any claims to their superiority, he says that "there is no doubt that these shoes provide good flexibility and stability as well as excellent shock absorption." Copeland is a little more skeptical about the value of pumped-up Reeboks. They provide excellent ankle support, he says, but a good lacing system is probably equally effective.

And some professionals dismiss these innovations completely. "They're all marketing gimmicks," says Andrea Cracchiolo, M.D., an orthopedic surgeon who is director of the University of California at Los Angeles Foot and Ankle Clinic. For the average weekend athlete, "most athletic shoes in the $50 range are quite acceptable."

Ultimately it's up to you—and your pocketbook. Some of these shoes are extraordinarily expensive, costing as much as $200. If you're a dedicated athlete, not just a weekend player, they may be worth the tab.

Q: What makes a good tennis shoe?

A: For tennis and other racket sports, you want a shoe that's as lightweight as a running shoe but that "gives" enough for quick side-to-side sliding. (Running shoes, which have too much traction, could cause a foot or ankle injury if used for tennis.) The sole beneath the ball of the foot should be flexible, allowing repeated, quick, forward movements. On soft courts (clay, grass), wear a softer-soled shoe that allows better traction, with a flat tread to prevent clay or grass clogs. On hard courts, you can wear a sole with greater—that is, a nubbier—tread.

To prevent a subungual hematoma, or tennis toe, the toe box should be more padded than it is in a running shoe; the heel should also be padded and snug-fitting to prevent slipping from side to side. Uppers should be made of leather, nylon mesh or canvas.

Q: I suppose sports like football and basketball require a very different type of shoe?

A: That's right. With those sports, the priority is to reduce the risk of traumatic injury. And of course, professional football and baseball players—and even some youngsters who play those sports—also wear cleats for traction.

- **Basketball, volleyball.** Basketball shoes should be of heavier-weight leather, with a thick, stiff rubber sole ridged for traction on wood floors. High-tops provide support when landing from a jump and help prevent ankle sprains. There should be extra cushioning in the midsoles and ankle area. Basketball players give their shoes such a pounding, says the APMA, that a player who wears his shoes for five days of play a week should replace them every two to three months. Volleyball shoes are similar to basketball shoes but tend to be lighter and have less midsole support and a crepe or rubber sole that allows for quick starts and stops.

- *Football, soccer, lacrosse.* Because they improve traction, cleats are the footwear of choice for all contact sports. However, cleats can also be a source of irritation, because much of the weight is carried on the small areas of the shoe sole where the cleats are attached. Cleats should be light and flexible and always fit properly, or else they increase the risk of ankle injuries. (Cleats come in different materials—rubber, plastic—and sizes for different playing surfaces.) At least a finger's width should separate the tip of the big toe and the end of the shoe. Shoes for contact sports should be leather, for protection, and tightly laced.

- *Baseball.* The observations about cleats, above, also apply to baseball. In some competitive baseball leagues, however, players wear shoes with metal spikes instead. Like cleats, spikes require a period of adjustment; if you're not used to them, you can twist your ankle more easily than you would in a pair of running shoes. Above all, be careful to avoid hurting other players. Don't wear shoes with either cleats or spikes off the field. Baseball shoes have nylon mesh and leather uppers.

Q: Are special shoes required for other sports such as bicycling and golf?

A: That depends on how aggressively you participate in those sports.

A cycling shoe must have a stable **shank**—the part of the sole between the heel and the ball—to efficiently transfer power from your feet to the pedals. If you wear sneakers without a shank support, your foot collapses through the arch when you pedal; that can cause arch pain, tendon problems or a burning sensation on the soles of the feet. If you bike for leisure—that is, not competitively—and you don't have any particular foot problems, you can probably get all the support you need from a cross-training shoe, possibly adding a heel lift.

A good athletic shoe with arch support and cushioning is adequate for most golfers, as long as it complies with course rules. If you have the money and think you have the need, you might consider one of the high-tech golf shoes with a graphite shank reinforcement, which keeps them light and adds strength.

Q: What about skiing? Can I just go with the regular footwear that's sold or rented?

A: If you're talking about cross-country skiing, there is not much variety in footwear anyway, so your choice is limited. Compared with boots for downhill skiing, cross-country footwear is relatively simple and unstructured—more like the cycling shoe described above than like the rigid downhill ski boot. Cross-country boots should not irritate the balls of the feet or promote blisters.

On the other hand, downhill ski boots offer an almost dizzying array of choices, with systems of cables and buckles to perfect the fit. A snug fit is particularly important because of the risk of injury from the constant forward motion and lateral movement of skiing.

If you have structural problems such as flat feet (or even, sometimes, if you don't), you may have noticed that when you ski downhill, you have a tendency to "edge"— that is, your foot and ski roll to the inside or outside edge. This reduces your control going down the slopes, slows you down and—most worrisome—puts a lot of pressure on your knees. Increasingly, ski shops are promoting something called "skithotics"—orthotics that hold the foot in a neutral position.

Q: Any guidelines for ice skates?

A: Like ski boots, ice skates should fit snugly. If skates are too loose, your muscles will tighten,

which could lead to painful spasms; also, loose skates
don't provide proper ankle support. Skates that are too
big or too small may cause blisters, inflammation or
nail irritation.

To ensure a snug fit, lace your skates all the way up.
If you have side-to-side wobbling in the heel area, which
is common, you can usually correct this with "shims," or
pads, in the heel. Shims can also be added to the middle
of the skate for a snugger fit.

Q: What about athletic shoes for children?

A: For children under the age of 10, an all-purpose
athletic shoe works well for most sports. However, avoid using a running shoe for activities that involve
lateral movement, such as tennis, because it may increase
the risk of injury. After the age of 10, when the child's
feet are more formed and he can play more competitively, he should have shoes that are designed for his
particular sport, if possible.

If your child is lobbying hard for one of those pricey
pairs of shoes, spend the money instead on two pairs
of less expensive shoes. They're often just as good,
and it's better to have a second pair so you can rotate
the shoes, saving on wear and letting them dry out
between games.

Q: Is there anything else I need to know about athletic shoes?

A: As we've indicated in the discussion of skithotics, athletes often need orthotics or pedorthics in addition to the appropriate athletic shoe for their particular sport. If your feet are flat or arched or you tend to develop shinsplints, you may require specially designed inlays, removable pads that act as additional shock absorbers. Most athletic shoes are manufactured with inlays. You or a professional can replace that with one tailored to your particular needs. For a discussion of orthotics, see chapter 5.

But in our focus on shoes, it's important not to lose sight of the fact that proper footwear is only part of an athlete's armament. Before you embark on a sport, you should prepare your legs and feet with a series of stretching exercises. To avoid Achilles tendinitis and plantar fasciitis, for example, runners and cross-country skiers need to loosen up their muscles before they set out. Shoes can take you only so far; you have to do the rest.

5 PREVENTION

Q: How can I prevent foot problems?

A: As we've explained in previous chapters, the best way to prevent—or at least mitigate—foot problems is to wear appropriate shoes. While chapter 4 focused on athletic footwear, in this chapter we offer guidelines for selecting any type of footwear, for the office as well as the field. In addition, we discuss various types of orthotics, traditionally known as orthoses—shoe inserts designed to correct or minimize existing structural problems and prevent further problems.

But shoes that fit correctly aren't the only means of treating your feet well. As discussed in this chapter, exercise, massage and regular care—using products found in virtually every medicine chest and kitchen—can also help you maintain healthy feet.

PROPER FOOTWEAR

Q: How should I choose a shoe?

A: Here are 10 tips on proper shoe fit from the American Orthopaedic Foot and Ankle Society (AOFAS), the National Shoe Retailers Association and the Pedorthic Footwear Association:

"1. Sizes vary among shoe brands and styles. Don't select shoes by the size marked inside the shoe. Judge the shoe by how it fits your foot.

2. Select a shoe that conforms as nearly as possible to the shape of your foot.

3. Have your feet measured regularly. The size of your feet changes as you grow older.

4. Have *both* feet measured. Most people have one foot larger than the other. Fit to the larger foot.

5. Fit at the end of the day when your feet are their largest. (Feet stretch and spread, and sometimes swell, during the day.)

6. Stand during the fitting process and check that there is adequate space (⅜ to ½ inch) for your longest toe at the end of each shoe.

7. Make sure the ball of your foot fits comfortably into the widest part (ball pocket) of the shoe.

8. Don't purchase shoes that feel too tight, expecting them to 'stretch' to fit.

9. Make sure your heel fits comfortably in the shoe with a minimum amount of slippage.

10. Walk in the shoe to make sure it fits and feels right. (Fashionable shoes *can* be comfortable!)''

Q: Sounds like I shouldn't buy shoes from mail-order catalogs. Is that true?

A: Not necessarily. As long as you follow the fitting suggestions listed above, there's no reason that you should not order shoes from a catalog. When your shoes arrive, wear them around the house, preferably on carpeting to keep them scuff-free. If there's a problem with the fit, you can always return them.

One way to improve your odds of getting well-fitting shoes sight unseen is to stay with one or two manufacturers. Size and fit vary from one manufacturer to another because each is working with a different series of lasts— the model of a foot over which shoes are shaped. So if you usually take a size 8 in a certain make, it's probably safe to order that shoe by mail. Still, even individual shoes have slight variations, so when you receive the shoes, test them for proper fit.

Q: Fit aside, are there other standards I should use in buying a shoe?

A: There are a number of things to look for in a well-made shoe. These include a sole that absorbs shock well (leather may be haute couture, but it's usually too thin to offer much protection), an insole that cushions and an upper that breathes (vinyl and urethane are cheaper, but leather *is* better here). In her book *My Feet Are Killing Me!,* podiatrist Suzanne M. Levine offers the following considerations:

- A good shoe often has a rigid shank of steel, wood or leather beneath the arch for support. Check to see if the midsole of the shoe is flexible; if so, it won't be very supportive.

- Look for shoe construction in which the sole and the upper are sewn to a rib or welt of material (often leather) rather than sewn directly together.

- Check the back and sides of the shoe for a counter, the piece of stiff material that adds heel support.

- Run your hand along the inside lining to find possible irritants—loose linings, wrinkles, lasting tacks or any ridges between the sole and sides.

- Make sure the stitching is neat. No loose threads or missed stitches! Stress points should be double-stitched.

Q: Any advice specifically for women?

A: Doctors who take care of the feet have a lot of "don'ts" for women—especially, don't wear spike or stiletto heels. Stilettos, which elevate the heel 4 to 5 inches, aggravate every foot problem associated with high-fashion shoes—bunions, hammertoes, calluses, neuromas, Achilles tendinitis—and can also cause back pain from the tilted pelvis and unstable posture created by these shoes.

"With stilettos, each step is a controlled fall," says Carol Frey, M.D., an orthopedic surgeon at the University of Southern California and director of the Orthopaedic Foot and Ankle Center, Orthopaedic Hospital, Los Angeles. She adds that stilettos have even been implicated in auto accidents in which heels got caught in brakes and car carpeting.

In fact, many foot specialists say, don't wear any heel that's more than 1 inch high—and preferably only ½ inch.

Q: So that means wearing "sensible"—that is, dowdy—shoes all the time?

A: Fortunately, the choice isn't that limited. There are attractive low-heeled shoes. And while 4-inch spikes are taboo, foot specialists say it's OK to wear 3-inch heels occasionally for short distances, such as walking from a car to a restaurant. "Treat high heels as treats," advises Enyi Okereke, M.D., an orthopedic surgeon at the University of Pennsylvania Medical Center, in Philadelphia. That applies to stilettos, as well as clunky high heels.

Q: Any special guidance for children's shoes?

A: For fitting children's shoes, AOFAS offers guidelines that are very similar to the points enumerated above for adults. In addition, it cautions that to accommodate growth and provide "wiggle room," you should allow a thumb's width from the end of the longest toe to the end of the shoe. Children should be measured for shoe size at every store visit because their feet can grow very rapidly.

Babies and crawlers do not need shoes, only soft booties or socks to keep their feet warm. When toddlers wear shoes, they should be lightweight with smooth soles so that the shoe doesn't grab on to the floor, causing the child to tumble. High-tops are acceptable, but they're not necessary for ankle support.

Above all, AOFAS and other professional associations caution that children should not wear hand-me-down shoes. Because young feet are so malleable, children can easily pick up each other's structural problems.

Q: How long should I wear the same pair of shoes?

A: That depends on a number of factors, including how hard you wear your shoes and how often you change them. Foot specialists advise people to have a few pairs of shoes and rotate their use; that way, each pair has a chance to air out between wearings. You can also extend the life of your shoes by treating them well—for example, using shoe and boot trees to retain their shape.

Above all, maintain the heels. Run-down heels can result in uneven walking patterns and poor posture and, ultimately, can shorten the life of the shoe. Men often suffer from overused footwear with worn heels and no support. "Men tend to wear shoes until they're dead," says Frey. Have a shoemaker put a tip on a worn heel.

Q: **Why don't these professional organizations endorse certain footwear in the same way that the American Dental Association endorses toothpaste?**

A: They do, but the endorsements aren't emblazoned on shoe boxes the way they are on tubes of toothpaste. A couple of years ago, AOFAS undertook an ambitious program to conduct what it called the "first-ever scientifically based evaluation of shoewear," based on a detailed laboratory analysis of 14 different shoe components. Unfortunately, most manufacturers dragged their feet, and AOFAS dropped its plans.

The American Podiatric Medical Association (APMA) does award a Seal of Acceptance to a wide variety of shoes and shoe-related products, and AOFAS recently endorsed some shoes. But these endorsements don't seem to get played up. With a few exceptions—notably Rockport, which makes the sort of street shoes that foot specialists love—the shoe manufacturers want to preserve their independence.

Do It Yourself: A Self-Care Kit for Your Feet

Every home medicine chest—and kitchen cabinet—should have a few products that are useful for keeping feet healthy and reasonably attractive. (It's debatable whether, despite the commercial claims of some products, anything can make adult feet pretty!) Below, we list these standard items and their applications. The list does not include the many over-the-counter treatments, which are discussed in chapter 2, for corns, calluses, athlete's foot and other common foot problems.

- *Toenail clippers.* Use to trim toenails straight across, preventing ingrown nails.

- *File or emery board.* Use to file down nails after clipping.

- *Orange stick or hindu stick.* Use to push back cuticles, the tissue adjacent to the nail.

- *Talcum powder or cornstarch.* Apply regularly—daily or more often as needed—to feet and shoes, to absorb moisture.

- *Rubbing alcohol.* Rub on feet to ease cramps (discussed in chapter 4) and cool off sweaty feet.

- *Moisturizers.* Apply to feet regularly, particularly during the dry winter months. Ointments such as petroleum jelly are best for keeping skin moist. Because these tend to be greasy and stain, however, many people prefer creams and lotions, which must be applied more often. Creams and lotions are equally effective as moisturizers. Active ingredients should include vegetable oils, mineral oils and lanolin, although the latter may provoke a rash or other allergic reaction in some people.

- *Petroleum jelly.* Apply to brittle nails daily.

- *Pumice stone.* Rub on calluses and dry skin to remove dead skin. A pumice stone—a rough-edged stone you can buy in most drugstores—is arguably as effective as any of the high-priced over-the-counter buffing creams.

- *Tea bags, baking soda (sodium bicarbonate), kosher salt.* Add these to water for homemade remedies for sweaty, smelly feet. A solution of very weak tea (a pail of warm water with three tea bags) provides enough tannic acid to soothe the feet and reduce perspiration; kosher salt in water (about ½ cup of salt per quart of water) also helps. A foot soak with baking soda (1 tablespoon in 1 quart of luke-warm water) increases the skin's acidity, helps prevent fungal or bacterial infections and reduces odor.

ORTHOTICS

Q: **Is orthotics just a fancy name for orthopedic shoes?**

A: Not at all. In fact, the so-called orthopedic shoe— that clunky oxford shoe with arch support that may have been worn by your grandmother a couple of decades ago—is a misnomer: According to Glenn Copeland, D.P. M., author of *The Foot Book,* there was nothing particularly orthopedic about it. (Technically an oxford shoe is a stout, low shoe that laces over the instep.) In any event, the orthopedic shoe has largely disappeared, displaced by athletic shoes that generally provide better stability, shock absorption and flexibility than those oxfords.

The other misconception is that orthotics are only arch supports. Although that's often the case, orthotics may be inserted anywhere in the shoe to make standing, walking and running more comfortable and efficient, generally by altering slightly the angles at which the feet strike the ground. Although people generally do not need orthotics unless they have already developed a foot problem, orthotics are also used to prevent further problems from occurring.

Q: How do I know whether I need orthotics or just a different shoe?

A: If you're uncertain or you're having chronic problems, you should consider consulting a podiatrist or orthopedic surgeon who specializes in the foot and ankle. If a foot care specialist thinks orthotics are in order, he'll measure you for them—either by taking a foam or plaster impression of your foot or, increasingly, by using a computerized "gait analysis" that shows how you're distributing your weight.

Based on that information, the foot care specialist may write a prescription for custom-made orthotics that you can have filled by an orthotics manufacturer or pedorthist. Foot specialists aren't the only ones to write such prescriptions, by the way; a pregnant woman with foot problems could get a prescription from her obstetrician, for example.

Q: If I can get a prescription for orthotics, does that mean my insurance carrier will pay for it?

A: That depends on your insurer and your reason for getting orthotics. As noted in chapter 3, people with diabetes are generally covered for foot treatment, including orthotics. And there's a good chance that Medicare will cover part of the cost of orthotics for Medicare beneficiaries. But if you're a runner who's buying arch supports for your plantar fasciitis, don't expect your private insurer to reimburse you.

Q: OK, back to orthotics themselves.
What are they like?

A: Depending on their precise purpose, orthotics take a variety of shapes and forms and are constructed from any of some 200 different compounds, including high-tech materials such as graphite and silastic.

Probably the best-known orthotics are arch supports— removable inlays that run the length of the shoe, from heel to ball or toe, and that support and protect the arch. Arch supports can be soft and compressible, semirigid (a classic model is a lamination of leather and cork) or rigid (made out of plastic, leather or another firm— but never uncomfortable—material). The advantage of rigid arch supports is that they last longer and don't change shape.

Q: I know some orthotics provide arch support. But what else can they do?

A: Orthotics can correct a variety of structural problems of the foot. To relieve pain from a heel spur, for example, a foot specialist might prescribe an orthotic designed as a relatively soft, horseshoe- or doughnut-shaped pad that redistributes over a wider area the weight that ordinarily lies on the heel. The spur, in effect, floats in the air. Or for chronic ankle pain and instability, the orthotic would be a foot balancer inside the shoe, made of a semirigid material, to take the stress off the injured side of the ankle and redistribute the body's weight.

Soft orthotic devices, which take pressure off uncomfortable or sore spots, are particularly good for people with diabetes or arthritis whose feet have become badly deformed. They're also helpful when people have lost much of the protective fatty tissue on the side of the foot. However, because soft orthoses tend to be bulkier, you may need to buy larger shoes or have your shoes modified.

Q: Is that where pedorthists come in?

A: That's one example. Pedorthists do get involved in modifying shoes to accommodate orthotics. But pedorthists also make changes to the shoe to improve fit and balance. To relieve fallen arches, for example, a pedorthist might apply to the sole of the shoe no fewer than three corrective devices: a Thomas heel, a comma-shaped bar and a transverse bar. The Thomas heel, a wedge-shaped heel slightly longer than a normal heel, changes the balance of a person's heel and exerts a twisting force on the bones of his arch; this makes the toes turn inward, correcting the ducklike gait seen in many people with fallen arches. The comma-shaped bar, near the middle of the sole, supports the arch, while the transverse bar, across the ball of the sole, supports the metatarsals.

For people who have difficulty walking due to arthritis, pedorthists could make other external modifications— flares, wedges and elevations—to stabilize the foot. Pedorthists may also modify the interior of the shoe, as well as the exterior.

To locate a pedorthist, ask your podiatrist or other foot care specialist or contact the Pedorthic Footwear Association, listed on page 163.

Q: Don't children sometimes wear orthotics?

A: Yes, for certain congenital foot deformities. If, for example, children truly do have collapsed arches (and not the seemingly flat feet characteristic of most babies) or arches that are abnormally high, it may be possible to correct either condition with orthotics. Most foot specialists recommend that children with such deformities wear orthoses soon after they start walking, to enable their bones to grow in as normal a position as possible.

As a rule, foot care specialists prescribe rigid orthotics for children. These typically need to be replaced frequently to accommodate the foot as it grows and changes shape. How long children need to wear orthotics depends on how significant their problems are.

Q: Aren't some orthotics sold in drugstores?

A: In addition to all the callus and corn pads and moleskins mentioned in chapter 2, drugstores are increasingly selling some of the more widely used orthotic devices over the counter. Although orthotists

and pedorthists might object to their inclusion as orthotics because they're not custom-made, here are the most common devices:·

- *Heel cup.* Made of plastic or rubber, the heel cup is designed to give support around the heel while providing relief from pressure on tender areas. The heel cup, like the prescription "doughnut," can be an effective way to alleviate pain beneath the heel caused by plantar fasciitis or heel spurs.

- *Arch support.* Made of many types of materials, the arch support can be placed in a shoe after removing the standard insole that comes with most shoes. Arch supports can help support weak arches, as well as provide extra shock absorbency, but choose your product with care: The foam over-the-counter arch supports often don't hold up for very long, while the so-called spring arch supports, made of metal, are often uncomfortable to wear.

- *Metatarsal pad.* Made of felt or firm rubber, the pad—which has adhesive on its flat side—is applied to the insole beneath the ball of the foot to relieve pressure on that area. It can help alleviate pain beneath the area near the big toe (if the problem is sesamoiditis, an inflammation that often follows a stress fracture in either of the two small sesamoid bones) or near the other toes (if the problem is metatarsalgia, an inflammation of the metatarsal bones and their soft tissue sheath, often caused by high-heeled shoes).

Q: Are custom-made orthotics any better than the over-the-counter variety?

A: That depends, as usual, on whom you ask. According to Andrea Cracchiolo, M.D., director of the University of California at Los Angeles Foot and Ankle Clinic, "Over-the-counter ones costing $50 are probably as good" as custom-made orthotic inserts, which can cost as much as $1,000 a pair.

But other foot specialists swear by custom-made orthotics. Copeland, for example, compares buying direct-mail orthotics from nonmedical suppliers to ordering prescription contact lenses by mail. He maintains that it's important that a licensed practitioner take a measure of your foot, just as an eye care professional needs to fit the lens to your eye. Ultimately the decision is yours—or your foot's.

EXERCISE

Q: Are there any exercises designed for the feet?

A: In moderation, the best exercise you can give your feet is to walk on them. Walking contributes to your general health (and thus indirectly to the well-being of your feet)—it strengthens your heart and lungs, helps control weight and high blood pressure, improves muscle tone in your legs and abdomen, reduces arthritis pain and slows osteoporosis. And as mentioned in chapter 4, compared with running, walking carries a significantly lower risk of injury, as long as you're wearing good shoes that fit well. Walking subjects your feet and ankles to less wear and tear than any other exercise, with the exception of swimming.

Walking aside, a number of exercises are designed specifically for the feet. In 1997, for example, the AOFAS Heel Pain Study Group reported that keeping to a daily regimen of simple stretching exercises was very effective in treating heel pain.

The AOFAS study divided 236 people with heel pain into five separate groups. One group did only plantar fascia and Achilles tendon-stretching exercises. The other four groups used either an over-the-counter shoe insert or a custom-made arch support along with the stretching exercises. After eight weeks of treatment, 72 percent of those who did only Achilles tendon and plantar fascia stretching felt that their condition had improved. Of those who used an insert or arch support as well as exercise, up to 95 percent said their condition had improved.

Glenn B. Pfeffer, M.D., a San Francisco orthopedic surgeon who was the principal author of the study, said exercise could mean relief for women who regularly wear high-heeled shoes.

Q: What do these stretching exercises involve?

A: One exercise that will help loosen the Achilles tendon is a simple "sprinter's stretch." Lean against a wall, with your arms outstretched and your

palms pressed against the wall at shoulder height. Keep
one knee straight while you bend the other knee and
push into the wall. Try to keep both heels flat on the
ground as you slowly lean forward into the bent knee.
When you feel the arch of your foot stretch, hold the
position for 10 seconds, then relax and straighten up.
Repeat this exercise 20 times for each heel.

Another simple exercise is to hold on to a table, chair
or countertop and flex both knees as you slowly squat.
Try to keep both heels on the ground as long as you can
on the way down. You will feel the arches of your feet
stretch as your heel finally starts to rise off the ground
during the squat. When you feel these muscles really
stretching, hold that position 10 seconds, then straighten
up. Repeat this exercise 20 times.

Q: **Since so many foot problems involve the toes, are there any exercises specifically for toes?**

A: Yes—and they're not for ballerinas only!
Here's a toe-strengthening program, devised
by orthopedic surgeon Carol Frey:

- *Toe raise, toe point, toe curl.* Hold each position
  for five seconds. Repeat 10 times. Recommended
  for people with hammertoes or toe cramps.

- *Toe squeeze.* Place small corks between your
  toes and squeeze for five seconds. Repeat 10 times.
  Recommended for people with hammertoes or
  toe cramps.

- *Big toe pull.* Place a thick rubber band around the big toes, and pull them away from each other, toward the small toes. Hold for five seconds. Repeat 10 times. Recommended for people with bunions or toe cramps.

- *Toe pull.* Put a thick rubber band around all of your toes and spread them. Hold this position for five seconds. Repeat 10 times. Recommended for people with bunions, hammertoes or toe cramps.

- *Golf ball roll.* Roll a golf ball back and forth under the ball of your foot for two minutes. Recommended for people with plantar fasciitis, arch strain or foot cramps.

- *Towel curl.* Place a small towel on the floor and curl your toes around it to bring it toward you. You can increase the resistance by putting a weight on the end of the towel. Relax and repeat this exercise five times. Recommended for people with hammertoes, toe cramps or pain in the ball of the foot.

- *Marble pickup.* Place 20 marbles and a small bowl on the floor. Using your toes, pick up one marble at a time and put it in the bowl. Do this exercise until you have picked up all 20 marbles. Recommended for people with pain in the ball of the foot, hammertoes or toe cramps.

- *Sand walking.* Whenever you have the opportunity, take off your shoes and walk in the sand at the beach. This not only massages the feet, but it also strengthens the toes. Recommended for general foot conditioning.

Q: Any other foot care tips?

A: A soak in hot water and Epsom salts at the end of the day, followed by a massage, can be wonderfully therapeutic for tired, aching feet. "The heat is terrific for getting the blood going and relaxing the muscles," says New York podiatrist Terry L. Spilken.

Then pamper your feet after the bath. Sitting on a mat, chair or bed, rotate each ankle clockwise and counterclockwise to loosen muscles. Next, moisturize: Put some moisturizer in the palm of one hand and rest one foot on the opposite knee. With the heel of your hand, knead your foot in a circular motion, from one end to the other. Knead the arch with your thumbs. Move along the soles and sides of your foot. Flex each toe back and gently rotate it. Tug it gently. Switch feet and repeat.

Q: Is there anything else I should do for my feet?

A: As noted in earlier chapters, don't smoke: It impairs the circulation of blood to your feet. If you exercise regularly, control your diet and follow the prescriptives offered in this chapter, you should be able to keep your best foot forward!

APPENDIX

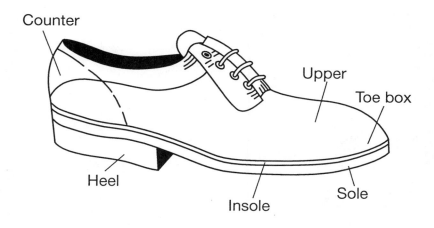

The Anatomy of a Shoe

INFORMATIONAL
AND
MUTUAL-AID GROUPS

American Academy of Podiatric Sports Medicine
1729 Glastonberry Rd.
Potomac, MD 20854
800-438-3355
301-424-7440

American Diabetes Association
1660 Duke St.
Alexandria, VA 22314
800-232-3472
800-342-2383
www.diabetes.org

American Orthopaedic Foot and Ankle Society
1216 Pine St., Suite 201
Seattle, WA 98101
800-235-4855
206-223-1120
Fax: 206-223-1178
E-mail: aofas@aofas.org
www.aofas.org

American Orthotics and Prosthetics Association
1650 King St., Suite 500
Alexandria, VA 22314
703-836-7116
Fax: 703-836-0838
E-mail: info@theaopa.org
www.theaopa.org/

American Podiatric Medical Association
9312 Old Georgetown Rd.
Bethesda, MD 20814-1698
800-FOOTCARE (800-366-8227)
301-571-9200
E-mail: askapma@apma.org
www.apma.org

Arthritis Foundation
1330 W. Peachtree St.
Atlanta, GA 30309
800-283-7800
404-872-7100
www.arthritis.org

National Aging Information Center
330 Independence Ave., S.W., Room 4656
Washington, DC 20201
800-222-2225
202-619-7501
Fax: 202-401-7620
E-mail: naic@ban-gate.aoa.dhhs.gov
www.aoa.dhhs.gov/naic

Pedorthic Footwear Association
9861 Broken Land Pkwy., Suite 255
Columbia, MD 21046-1151
800-673-8447
410-381-7278
Fax: 410-381-1167
E-mail: info@cpeds.org
www.cpeds.org

Wound Care Institute, Inc.
1541 N.E. 167th St.
North Miami Beach, FL 33162
305-919-9192
E-mail: Tamara@woundcare.org
www.woundcare.org

GLOSSARY

Achilles tendon: The large tendon at the back of the lower leg that inserts into the back of the heel.

Arthrodesis: The surgical fusion of the subtalar (below the ankle) joint.

Arthroscope: A flexible viewing tube, about the diameter of a pencil, that provides the surgeon with an inside view of the joint. Arthroscopic surgery is often used in the treatment of arthritic feet and ankles.

Athlete's foot: A skin disease, technically known as *tinea pedis,* that is caused by a fungus and most often occurs between the toes.

Blister: A fluid-filled sac that often forms between the top layers of the skin of the feet, usually as the result of the skin rubbing against shoes.

Bromhidrosis: Foot odor, typically caused by decomposition of bacteria that live on the skin.

Buerger's disease: A circulatory syndrome, occurring mainly in men under the age of 40, that leads to cold and numb feet. In some cases, it can progress to tissue necrosis and gangrene.

Bunion: A bony bump on the base of the big toe that may occur when one toe overlaps another.

Bunionette: A protuberance of bone at the outside of the foot behind the fifth (small) toe; also known as a tailor's bunion.

Bursa: One of the sacs of fluid that overlies and protects each joint of the body, including those in the toes.

Bursitis: Painful inflammation of a bursa.

Calcaneal bursitis: Inflammation of a bursa just under the weight-bearing surfaces of the heel bone; also known as policeman's heel.

Calcaneus: The heel bone; also the largest bone in the foot.

Callus: A thickened area of skin that forms in response to excessive pressure or friction, typically occurring on the ball of the foot, the heel or the underside of the big toe.

Charcot foot: A fracture or dislocation of the foot or ankle that sometimes occurs in people with diabetes, particularly if they also have peripheral neuropathy.

Claw toe: A deformity related to the hammertoe, in which a middle toe curls under rather than flexing (as it does in the hammertoe).

Clubfoot: A complicated congenital deformity in which the rearfoot is extremely flexed, with the forefoot going downward and inward.

Corn: A usually hard, yellowish circle of skin that forms on the surface of a toe in response to excessive pressure or friction. However, some corns—typically found between toes—are soft.

Counter: The part of a shoe that wraps around the heel.

Debridement: A procedure used to treat fungal nails and other infections in which the area is scraped free of diseased debris and treated with topical antifungals or antibiotics.

Distal osteotomy: One of two basic techniques used to cut and realign the first metatarsal and to eliminate a bunion. In this procedure, the far end of the bone is cut and moved laterally, reducing the angle between the first and second metatarsal bones.

Fibula: The outer and smaller of the two bones of the leg below the knee. The fibula connects with the tibia and the talus to form the ankle joint.

Flat feet: Feet with low arches—a condition created by an abnormal alignment of bones, an excessive elasticity of the ligaments or a muscle imbalance, or a combination of all three factors. Flat feet are usually not completely flat, although if the arches are sufficiently weak, they may eventually fall completely—a condition widely known as fallen arches.

Fracture: A break in a bone.

Frostbite: The freezing of body tissues due to overexposure to extreme cold. Typically this affects the extremities—the feet and hands.

Gangrene: Death of body tissues due to a loss of blood supply.

Gout: A form of arthritis that is caused by a buildup in the joints—typically, the big toe joints—of crystals of uric acid. Gout occurs most often in men who consume a rich diet.

Granuloma: A small benign tumor that sometimes forms along the nail margin when a toenail has become ingrown.

Haglund's deformity: Spurlike inflammation at the rear of the foot, between the heel bone and the Achilles tendon, that typically is caused by repetitive irritation from shoes with rigid heel counters.

Hallux: The big toe.

Hallux rigidus: A form of osteoarthritis in which the big toe becomes particularly stiff or rigid.

Hammertoe: A deformity involving a contracture of the toe, generally caused by a dropped metatarsal head and a tightening of the tendons that control toe movements.

Hyperhidrosis: Excessive sweating.

Ingrown toenail: A condition in which one or both corners or sides of a toenail curve and grow into the soft flesh of the toe, often leading to inflammation and infection.

Lateral: Referring to the outside of the foot.

Ligament: A thick, cordlike fiber that attaches bones to each other to keep them in correct alignment.

Mallet toe: A deformity, related to the hammertoe, in which the bent toe joint is the one near the tip, as opposed to the inside joint (as is the case with the hammertoe).

Matrix: The cells that grow the nail plate.

Medial: Referring to the inside of the foot.

Metatarsal: One of the five long bones that connect the tarsals in the midfoot to the phalanges, or bones in the toes.

Metatarsalgia: Painful inflammation of the metatarsal bones and their soft tissue sheaths.

Moleskin: A soft cloth made of sheep's wool that is used to reduce friction on blisters, bunions and calluses. An adhesive side allows the moleskin to stay in place in the shoe.

Morton's neuroma: A neuroma on the bottom of the foot between the toes that occurs when a small nerve to a toe becomes pinched between the toe joints and the shoe.

Mosaicplasty: A surgical technique in which small amounts of cartilage and bone are transplanted from the non-weight-bearing parts of the knee to the damaged talus.

Neurologist: A medical doctor specializing in the brain, spinal cord and peripheral nerves.

Neuroma: Swelling and inflammation of one or more nerves in the front part of the foot, typically between the third and fourth toes.

Nonsteroidal anti-inflammatory drug (NSAID): One of a group of drugs, including ibuprofen and many prescription drugs, having pain-relieving, fever-reducing and anti-inflammatory effects.

Nucleation: The deep-seated center of a corn or a callus.

Onychauxis: The thickening of the nails that often comes with age. Onychauxis may be caused by reduced circulation, which the elderly often develop, or by the small but repeated injuries that toenails suffer over the years.

Onychia: Inflammation of the nail matrix, the cells that grow the nail plate.

Onychogryposis: A condition, occurring primarily in the elderly, in which a nail thickens and curves into a ram's-horn shape.

Onycholysis: A condition in which a toenail plate begins to separate from the nail bed, generally after repeated injury or immersion in harsh chemicals.

Onychomadesis: A condition, common among runners, in which a toenail plate separates from the nail bed, beginning at the bottom of the nail. Onychomadesis may be caused by trauma, such as new running shoes that continually abrade the nail, in effect rubbing it off.

Onychomycosis: An infection of the bed and plate underlying the surface of a nail, caused by various types of fungi, that can also penetrate the nail; also known as ringworm.

Onychorrhexis: A condition, occurring primarily in the elderly, in which the nail splits longitudinally. The split can vary from a slight crack to nail-deep.

Orthopedist, or **orthopedic surgeon:** A medical doctor who specializes in treatment and surgery of the joints and related structures. Foot and ankle orthopedists have additional training in that area.

Orthotic, or **orthosis:** An arch support or other insert that is used to correct a structural problem of the foot or ankle. Orthotics protect the foot and improve the way it functions.

Orthotist: A specialist who provides custom-made orthotics. Unlike pedorthists, orthotists treat problems of the hip, spine and hands, as well as of the feet.

Osteochondritis dissecans (OCD): A deep bruise of the joint, involving the cartilage surface and underlying bone. OCDs often occur in athletes.

Osteoporosis: A condition, prevalent in the elderly, in which bones lose density and strength and are more susceptible to fracture.

Paronychia: Inflammation of the tissue adjacent to a toenail that is often caused by pedicures.

Pedorthist: A specialist who designs, manufactures, modifies and fits shoes and foot orthotics to alleviate foot problems caused by disease, overuse or injury.

Peripheral neuropathy: A gradual loss of nerve function in the extremities, primarily the feet, that is typically caused by diabetes.

Phalanx: One of the 14 bones that make up the toes.

Plantar fascia: The band of fibrous connective tissue that runs along the bottom of the foot and helps secure the arch.

Plantar fasciitis: Inflammation of the plantar fascia and one of the most common and painful causes of aching arches.

Plantar wart: A common infection, caused by viruses, that generally invades the sole of the foot through cuts and breaks in the skin.

Podiatrist: The primary specialist in foot care. Although not medical doctors, podiatric physicians (doctors of podiatric medicine, or D.P.M.'s) are licensed in all states to diagnose and treat—including surgically—conditions relating to the foot.

Pronation: The action of the arch in walking. In normal pronation, the arch lowers slightly when the heel comes to rest on the ground. In excessive pronation, the arch lowers too much, flattening to a point that it entirely touches the ground.

Proximal osteotomy: One of two basic techniques used to cut and realign the first metatarsal and to eliminate a bunion. In this procedure, the first metatarsal is cut at the near end of the bone.

Pump bump: See **Haglund's deformity**.

Purine: One of various protein compounds, found in organ meats, legumes and other foods, that can aggravate gout by elevating body levels of uric acid.

Raynaud's disease: A relatively common and minor circulatory disorder, occurring primarily in younger women, that results in cold and numb feet.

Reflexology: A form of alternative medicine that involves applying firm but gentle pressure to a particular part of the body—usually the soles of the feet. The object, however, is not to treat the feet themselves but instead to treat other body parts, including organs, muscles and bones, that reflexologists believe are directly linked to certain spots on the feet.

Reiter's syndrome: A group of arthritic conditions that may develop after an infection either in the bowel or in the urinary tract. Reiter's syndrome typically combines urethritis, arthritis and conjunctivitis (pinkeye), a common eye infection.

Sesamoid: Either of the two small bones that sit directly under the first metatarsal bone at the big toe joint.

Sesamoiditis: Painful inflammation of the area around the sesamoid bones.

Shank: The part of the sole of a shoe between the heel and the ball.

Shinsplints: Pain in the muscles of the lower leg, often caused by excessive pronation.

Spur: A spikelike calcium deposit, visible on x-rays, that forms on the heel or under a toe of the foot in response to trauma, sudden weight gain or other strain on a ligament, tendon or muscle.

Stress fracture: A break in a bone caused by sudden or repetitive stress. The difference between a stress fracture and other breaks is that, in a stress fracture, the bone is not displaced.

Subtalar joint: The joint where the talus and the calcaneus meet that allows rotation of the foot at the ankle.

Subungual hematoma: A condition in which blood accumulates under the nail, usually from accidental injury; also known as black-and-blue nail.

Supinated: Describing a foot with a comparatively high arch (as compared with a low-arched, or highly pronated, foot). If the foot is excessively supinated, it often absorbs shock poorly, leading to foot complications.

Talus: The anklebone.

Tarsal: One of the five irregular bones in the midfoot. Known collectively as the lesser tarsus, together these bones form the arch of the foot.

Tendinitis: Inflammation of a tendon.

Tendon: A strong band of tissue that connects muscle to bone.

Tenotomy: A minor surgical procedure used to correct hammertoes.

Tibia: The inner and larger of the two bones of the leg below the knee. The tibia connects with the fibula and the talus to form the ankle joint.

Toe box: The reinforced area in a shoe's tip that protects the foot.

Total contact cast: A special walking cast that allows a person to walk while foot sores heal by distributing the person's weight over the entire surface of the foot.

Vasoconstrictor: Any factor, typically a medication, that makes blood vessels constrict, reducing their ability to carry blood, particularly to the hands and feet.

Verruca: See **Plantar wart**.

SUGGESTED READING

Copeland, Glenn, D.P.M., with Stan Solomon. *The Foot Book: Relief for Overused, Abused & Ailing Feet.* New York: John Wiley & Sons, 1992.

Levine, Suzanne M., D.P.M. *50 Ways to Ease Foot Pain: Medical Book of Remedies.* New York: Penguin, 1995.

Levine, Suzanne M., D.P.M. *My Feet Are Killing Me!* New York: McGraw-Hill, 1987.

McGann, Daniel M., D.P.M., and L.R. Robinson. *The Doctor's Sore Foot Book.* New York: William Morrow, 1994.

Null, Gary, and Howard Robins. *How to Keep Your Feet and Legs Healthy for a Lifetime: The Only Complete Guide to Foot and Leg Care With Special Sections for Walkers, Joggers and Runners.* New York: Seven Stories Press, 1996.

Pritt, Donald S., D.P.M., and Morton Walker, D.P.M.
The Complete Foot Book: First Aid for Your Feet.
Garden City Park, N.Y.: Avery, 1996.

Tremaine, M. David, and Elias M. Awad. *The Foot & Ankle
Sourcebook: Everything You Need to Know.* Chicago:
Contemporary Books, 1996.

INDEX

Page numbers enclosed in brackets indicate illustrations.